# Demystifying Endometriosis

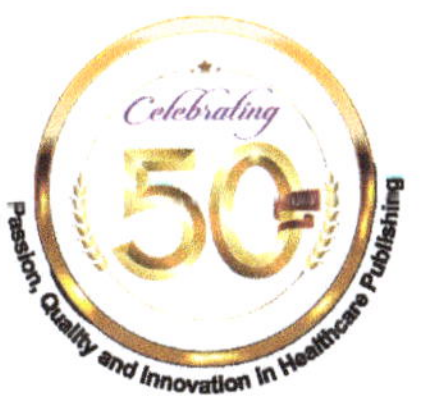

# Demystifying Endometriosis


**Kanthi Bansal** MD DGO FICOG
Director
Safal Fertility Foundation and Bansal Hospital
Ahmedabad, Gujarat, India


*Foreword*

Sameena Chowdhury

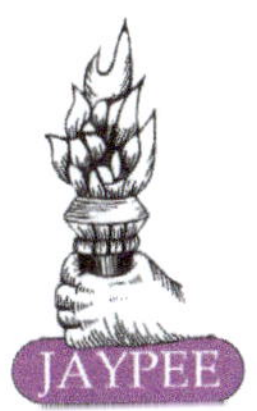


**JAYPEE BROTHERS MEDICAL PUBLISHERS**
*The Health Sciences Publisher*
New Delhi | London

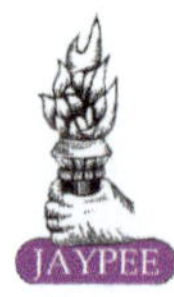 **Jaypee Brothers Medical Publishers (P) Ltd**

**Headquarters**

Jaypee Brothers Medical Publishers (P) Ltd
EMCA House, 23/23-B
Ansari Road, Daryaganj
New Delhi 110 002, India
Landline: +91-11-23272143, +91-11-23272703
+91-11-23282021, +91-11-23245672
E-mail: jaypee@jaypeebrothers.com

**Corporate Office**

Jaypee Brothers Medical Publishers (P) Ltd
4838/24, Ansari Road, Daryaganj
New Delhi 110 002, India
Phone: +91-11-43574357
Fax: +91-11-43574314
E-mail: jaypee@jaypeebrothers.com

**Overseas Office**

JP Medical Ltd
83 Victoria Street, London
SW1H 0HW (UK)
Phone: +44 20 3170 8910
Fax: +44 (0)20 3008 6180
E-mail: info@jpmedpub.com

Website: www.jaypeebrothers.com
Website: www.jaypeedigital.com



*Demystifying Endometriosis*

*First Edition*: **2021**

ISBN: 978-93-89776-39-3

**Dedicated to**

*My daughter-in-law, Divya Reddy Bansal*

# Contributors

**Anu Agarwal**  MBBS MD FIAMS
Senior Infertility Expert
Hysteroscopy and Laparoscopy Surgeon
Director
Vansh Fertility and Test Tube Baby Center
Ayushman Hospital and Trauma Center
Varanasi, Uttar Pradesh, India

**Anuradha Khanna**
MBBS MD FAMS FICS MNAMS FUICC FUWAI
Professor and Ex-Head
Department of Obstetrics and
Gynecology
Banaras Hindu University
Varanasi, Uttar Pradesh, India

**Apoorva Pallam Reddy**
MS DNB OBG Diploma in Gyne Endoscopy
Fellowship in Reproductive Medicine
Medical Director
Phoenix Speciality Clinic
Bengaluru, Karnataka, India

**Asha R Rao**  MD
Chief Consultant
Department of Infertility
RAO Hospital
Coimbatore, Tamil Nadu, India

**Ashish Kale**
MD (O & G) DNB MNAMS Dip. Endopelvic
Surgery (Germany) MICOG (India) FICS
Director
Asha IVF Center and Ashakiran Hospitals
(Pune, Jalna, Arunachal Pradesh)

**Astha Ubeja**  MBBS MD
Obstetrician and Gynecologist
Prakash Hospital and Research Centre
Khandwa, Madhya Pradesh, India

**Damodar R Rao**  MS
Associate Director and Senior Consultant
Department of Endogynecology
RAO Hospital
Coimbatore, Tamil Nadu, India

**Dhivya Sethuraman**  MD (O & G)
Associate Professor
Department of Obstetrics and
Gynecology
SRM Medical College-Hospital and
Research Centre
Tiruchirappalli, Tamil Nadu, India

**Gaurav S Desai**  MS FCPS
Assistant Professor
Obstetrics and Gynecology Pelvic
Surgeon Fertility Specialist
Seth GS Medical College and Kem
Hospital
Mumbai, Maharashtra, India

**Jaideep Malhotra**
MD FICOG FICMCH FICS FRCOG FMAS
Director
Global Rainbow Healthcare
Agra, Uttar Pradesh, India

**Kanthi Bansal**  MD DGO FICOG
Director
Safal Fertility Foundation and Bansal
Hospital
Ahmedabad, Gujarat, India

**Kriti Agarwal**  MD (O & G)
Junior Consultant
Care IVF
Kolkata, West Bengal, India

**Kuldeep Jain**  MD Fellow ART (Singapore)
IVF Consultant and Gynecology
Laparoscopic Surgeon
Director, KJIVF and Laparoscopy Center
New Delhi
Chairperson, Endometriosis Committee
New Delhi, India

**M Preethi**  MS
Resident Fellowship in Endogynecology
Department of Endogynecology
RAO Hospital
Coimbatore, Tamil Nadu, India

**Maansi Jain**
MS Fellowship in Reproductive Medicine and
Surgery (Singapore)
Consultant, ART
Department of Reproductive Medicine
KJIVF and Laparoscopy Center
New Delhi, India

**N Gayathri**  MD DNB (O & G)
Consultant Obstetrician and
Gynecologist
Shyamala Nursing Home
Tiruchirappalli, Tamil Nadu, India

**Narendra Malhotra**
MD FICMCH FICOG FRCOG FICS FMAS FIAP
President, INSARG
Past President, FOGSI/IFUMB/ISPAT/ISAR
Vice-President, WAPM/SAFOG
Professor
Sarajevo School of Science and
Technology, Croatia
Managing Director
Global Rainbow Health Care and
MNMH (P) Ltd
Agra, Uttar Pradesh, India

**Neharika Malhotra Bora**
MD (Gold Medalist) DRM (Germany) FICMCH
Fellow ICOG (Rep Med) ICOG (USG)
Joint Secretary, FOGSI
Chair, YTP Committee, FOGSI
Director and Consultant
Global Rainbow IVF and MNMH (P) Ltd
Agra, Uttar Pradesh, India

**Priyanka Honavar**  DNB
Assistant Professor
Department of Obstetrics and
Gynecology
Seth GS Medical College and Kem
Hospital
Mumbai, Maharashtra, India

**Rajeev Agarwal**  MBBS MD
Gynecologist and Infertility Specialist
Laparoscopic Surgeon and
Medical Director
Care IVF
Kolkata, West Bengal, India

**S Chitra**  MD DGO FICOG
Director, Consultant-Obstetrician,
Gynecologist and Infertility Specialist
Lalitha Nursing Home and
Janani Trichy Fertility Center
Tiruchirappalli, Tamil Nadu, India

**Sabita Dixit**  MBBS MS (O & G) MRCOG 1
Director, Dixit IVF Centre
Prayagraj, Uttar Pradesh, India

**Sameena Chowdhury**
MBBS MCPS FCPS FICS FICMCH DRH (UK)
FIAOG(IND)
President, Obstetrics and Gynecological
Society of Bangladesh (OGSB)
Professor
Central Hospital Ltd.
Dhaka, Bangladesh

**Sharmin Abbasi**
FCPS MCPS FMAS FACS (USA) MBBS
Associate Professor
Infertility Specialist and Gynecologist
Laparoscopic Surgeon
Department of Obstetrics and Gynecology
Anwer Khan Modern Medical
College-Hospital
Dhaka, Bangladesh

**Shikha Sachan**  MS (O & G)
Associate Professor
Department of Obstetrics and Gynecology
Banaras Hindu University
Varanasi, Uttar Pradesh, India

**Shyam V Desai**  MD DGO DFP MNAMS
President, Medical Director, Consultant
Endoscopic Surgeon, and
Laparoscopic Gynecologist
Mothercare Nursing Home
Mumbai, Maharashtra, India

**T Ramani Devi**  MD DGO FICS FICOG
Director
Consultant Obstetrician and Gynecologist
and Infertility Specialist
Ramakrishna Medical Centre LLP and
Janani Trichy Fertility Center
Trichy, Tamil Nadu, India

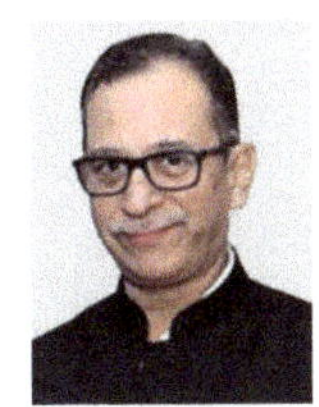

**Dr Anil Mehta**
President, AOGS

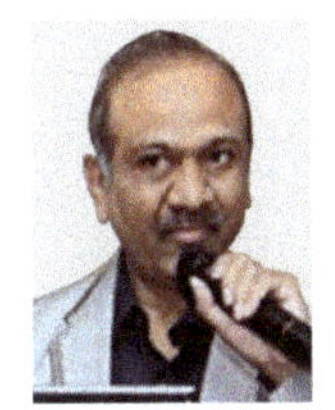

**Dr Mukesh Savaliya**
Secretary, AOGS

It gives us immense pleasure to inscribe message for the book *Demystifying Endometriosis*. Endometriosis is an enigma and so many women suffer from the pain of endometriosis and that affects the quality of their life. It is a great privilege for Ahmedabad Obstetrics and Gynecological Society (AOGS), Ahmedabad, Gujarat, India, as an organization that Dr Kanthi Bansal, one of its most valued; superior and knowledgeable member with renowned academic career, has penned a Demystifying Endometriosis. Dr Kanthi Bansal and the contributors to be congratulated for their innovative advocacy work for the women affected by the endometriosis.

On behalf of AOGS, we applaud her on publishing this tremendous book and highlighting the significance of management of endometriosis.

We wish her and her team all the best and congratulate her on this stupendous creation!

It is a matter of great pleasure for me to write foreword for the book of *"Demystifying Endometriosis"* published by Dr Kanthi Bansal. This book focused on the way that patients with endometriosis usually present and then proceeds to discuss the possible etiology, pathophysiology, management and recent updates. This will be more interesting and effective way of learning for the clinicians. 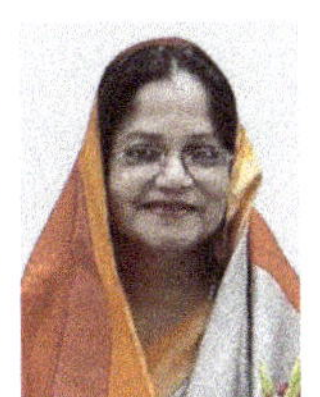

Endometriosis is a complex disease that affects a large number of women of reproductive age and imposes a significant burden on patients and society. In western populations, endometriosis is estimated to occur in 5 to 10% but the prevalence of endometriosis is suspected to be higher in Asian women, affecting approximately 15 to 20% of women. This prevalence can rise to 30 to 50% in women with infertility. Globally it is estimated that 176 million women are suffering with endometriosis. Among them most of the women have not been diagnosed and treated. It takes about 7 to 8 years delay to reach the final diagnosis. This suggested that an updated approach to determining the epidemiology of endometriosis in Asian populations is required to guide the patient care. This includes both the diagnosis and treatment of this debilitating condition.

Endometriosis is a common clinical situation which sometimes untreatable when primary objective is to treat infertility problem. In this book, it includes different chapters on endometriosis including, pathogenesis, diagnosis and staging, adolescent endometriosis, genesis of endometriosis, medical and surgical management, recurrent endometriosis, recent updates, endometriosis associated infertility and its management and new vision and past challenges of management of adenomyosis. This book is contributed by practical experience of passionate and knowledgeable gynecologist, ART specialist and scientists whose informative and concise chapters will help to navigate and guide to practice and to follow the right track and to upgrade themselves. The chapters regarding different aspects of endometriosis have been nicely elaborated in this book.

The understanding of the origins of pain associated with endometriosis is a priority for endometriosis research; such work should include specialists in the pain field and collaboration with the gynecologist. Because the most unbearable problem is pain and which destroy the quality-of-life of womanhood. This book focused on how to cure pain but more research is needed and recent updates need to implicate to reduce this pain.

There is a need for more well-designed, adequately powered, multicenter randomized controlled trials and long-term follow-up studies comparing different endometriosis treatment options against defined outcome measures.

I am extremely thankful to all the contributors for their caring and insightful write-ups and expert opinions. Without their assistance, this book could never be completed.

I hope this book will have wide acceptance and I will be very happy if the contents of this book fulfill the purpose for which the book has been written.

I congratulate to Dr Kanthi Bansal for taking a lead in publishing this book.

**Sameena Chowdhury**
MBBS MCPS FCPS FICS FIMCH DRH (UK)
Professor
President, Obstetrical and Gynecological Society of Bangladesh (OGSB)
Chairman, Endometriosis Committee, SAFOG

*"Not all scars show,*
*Not all wounds heal,*
*Not all illness can be seen,*
*Not all pain is obvious."*

Endometriosis is known as enigmatic disease. This condition poses various difficulties in the diagnosis and management. The main impact of this disease is pain and infertility. There are numerous books published on this subject but it is imperative to throw light on the latest consensus and development in this disease.

The book *Demystifying Endometriosis* consist of 12 chapters. The subject covers all aspects such as pathogenesis of endometriosis and its impacts, diagnosis and staging of endometriosis, adolescent endometriosis, management of pain in endometriosis, surgical management, newer molecules, recurrence and how to deal? infertility associated with endometriosis, endometrioma: diagnosis and management, deep infiltrating endometriosis, recent consensus in management of endometriosis and adenomyosis. The chapters include introduction, topic in its entirety, conclusion and references.

I truly believe that this book will be useful to postgraduates, medical fraternity at universities, medical collages and practicing clinicians. I sincerely hope that it will help in clearing many unknown important aspects of management of endometriosis and demystify this mysterious condition to our readers.

**Kanthi Bansal**

# Acknowledgments

This book is a culmination of the hard work of many individuals, who contributed in the book. I am indebted to each and every one of them for taking time from the midst of their hectic schedules and gave their contribution.

My special appreciation towards exceptional assistance and expertise of friends and colleagues from all over India. My sincere acknowledge and thanks to all those who contributed in various capacities to convert an idea into reality. I am extremely grateful to my family members for providing a warm back ground of love, encouragement and understanding that made this edition possible. Special thanks to Ms Shilpa Damodar, our scientific coordinator and Mr Ankit Talsania, our PRO for their sincere support in the compilation of this book.

I am are over helmed in all humbleness and gratefulness to acknowledge my depth to all those who have helped me to put these ideas, well above the level of simplicity and into something concrete.

I especially thankful to Shri Jitendar P Vij (Group Chairman), Mr Ankit Vij (Managing Director), Mr MS Mani (Group President), Ms Chetna Malhotra Vohra (Associate Director—Content Strategy), Ms Pooja Bhandari (Production Head), Ms Kritika Dua (Senior Development Editor) and the publishing staff at M/s Jaypee Brothers Medical Publishers (P) Ltd, New Delhi, India, for their work in completing this book successfully.

# Contents

# CHAPTER 1

# Pathogenesis and Impact of Endometriosis

*Ashish Kale*

## INTRODUCTION

Endometriosis is an extremely debilitating benign gynecological condition of women. It is commonly observed in the reproductive age.[1]

## DEFINITION

Histologically, it is defined as an abnormal implantation of endometrial tissues in ectopic locations outside the uterine cavity, primarily in the pelvic peritoneum, broad ligaments, ovaries, and rectovaginal septum.[2] Contemporary literature describes other less common sites, which include fallopian tubes, ureter, bladder, vagina, and pleura.[3]

Pathogenesis is described as the endometrial-like glands and stroma grows and undergoes cyclic proliferation and breaks down similar to the endometrium.[1] This internal bleeding that remains within the body results in local inflammation causing scar tissue formation.[1] The glandular cells within endometrium lodge cancer-associated mutations which are detected in ovarian cancers **(Fig. 1)**.[4]

Prevalence of endometriosis is as follows:

- 6–10% among all reproductive age group women
- 25–50% in infertile women
- 75–80% in women with chronic pelvic pain.[3]

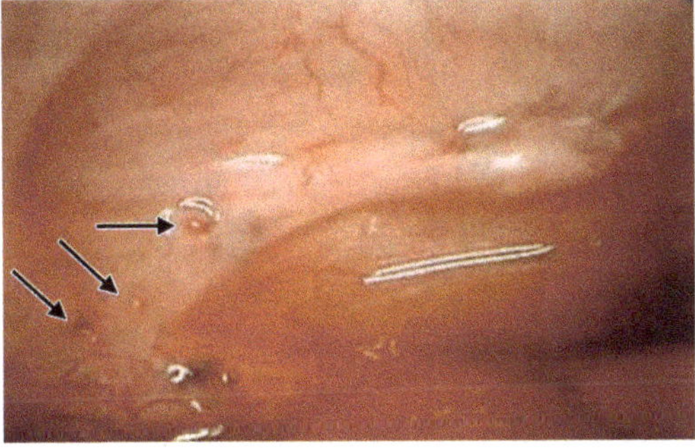

**Fig. 1:** Typical appearance of minimal endometriosis on the uterosacral ligaments.
*Source:* Davila GW (2018). What is the pathophysiology of endometriosis? [online] Available from: https://emedicine.medscape.com/article/271899-overview. [Last accessed March, 2020].

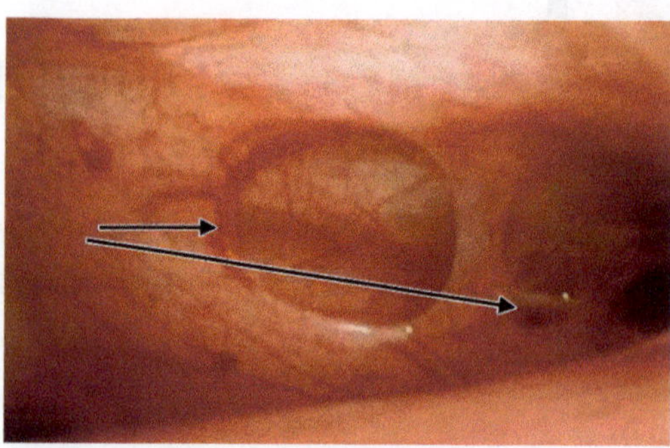

**Fig. 2:** Peritoneal erosions and adhesions in the posterior cul-de-sac. These are typical of more severe endometriosis.
*Source:* Davila GW (2018). What is the pathophysiology of endometriosis? [online] Available from: https://emedicine.medscape.com/article/271899-overview. [Last accessed March, 2020].

As compared to reproductive age group in women, the prevalence can reach up to 30–50% among symptomatic women.[5]

The prevalence of urinary tract endometriosis has been reported in the literature. To standardize the terminology, a classification of endometriosis has been proposed. It also helps to compare the outcomes of randomized studies in surgical treatment.[6]

Pelvic endometriosis is associated with adenomyosis with a prevalence of close to 90%. It accounts for infertility due to impaired uterine sperm transport.[7]

Impacts of endometriosis compromise the quality of life of affected women and also associate with dysmenorrhea, dysuria, and pain during defecation.[1]

According to previous studies, there are three forms of endometriosis in the pelvic cavity: peritoneal, ovarian, and deeply infiltrating lesions. The peritoneal and ovarian implants are described as white, red, and black colored, morphologically **(Fig. 2).**[1]

## PATHOGENESIS

There are several theories hypothesized for the pathophysiology of endometriosis which are as follows:

- Implantation theory
- Metaplasia theory
- Endometriosis disease theory
- Endometriosis as a stem cell-based condition.[1]

The most widely accepted hypothesis is that during menstruation, the endometrial cells are transported by retrograde flow of tissues intra-abdominally through fallopian tubes. It is assumed that a small lesion is established, which proliferates, differentiates, and invades leading to a progressive disease.[1] Retrograde menstruation is the most common physiological event, still it does not account for the implantation of endometrial tissues outside the uterine cavity.

There is another theory that reports heavier and continuous flow of menstruation with endometriosis increasing the material into pelvic cavity by retrograde reflux as compared to a healthy woman.[1]

In the adolescents, endometriosis is characterized by angiogenic and hemorrhagic peritoneal and ovarian lesions. And in the later stage, deep infiltrating endometriosis is developed.[8] One of the hypotheses explains that endometriotic cell has undergone genetic or epigenetic changes by radiation or dioxin and those changes develop deep endometriosis.[8]

Another theory, which is nonuterine in origin, is coelomic metaplasia theory. The coelomic epithelium gets transformed into endometrial-type tissues among women who have undergone total hysterectomy and also not taking estrogen replacement.[9]

Local inflammation and hyperactivation can be occurred if the fragment of endometrium does not get cleared out from the peritoneal cavity. Due to inflammation and hyperactivation, various compounds get secreted which can bring about metaplasia of the peritoneum or the development of the chocolate cyst of the ovary **(Fig. 3)**.[10]

The induction therapy proposes that unknown substances such as immunologic or hormonal factors shed from endometrium induce

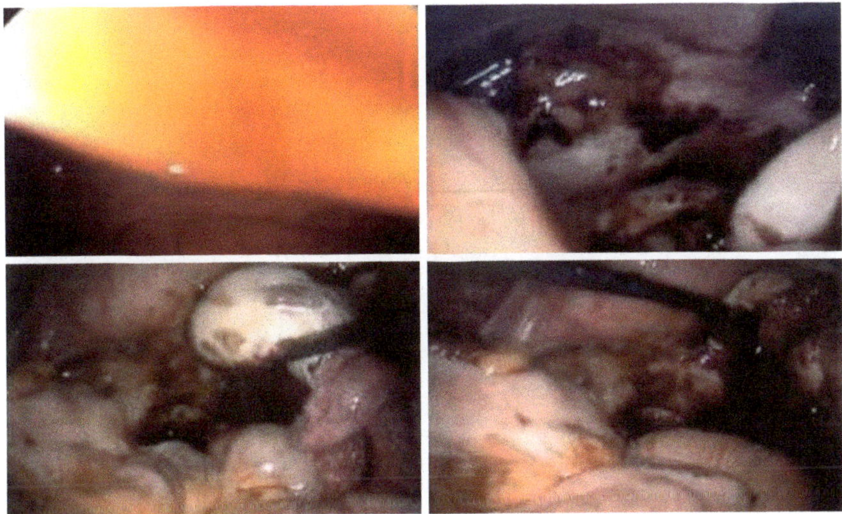

**Fig. 3:** Chocolate cyst of the ovary.
*Source:* Davila GW (2018). What is the pathophysiology of endometriosis? [online] Available from: https://emedicine.medscape.com/article/271899-overview. [Last accessed March, 2020].

endometrial-like tissues. Immunologic and hormonal dysfunctioning makes women susceptible for endometriosis disease.[1]

It is reported that endometriosis is a hormonal response that interprets the stimulation in steroid hormone production.[11]

## ETIOLOGY

- Early age of menarche
- Late menopause
- Delayed childbearing
- Shortened menstrual cycles
- Family history of endometriosis
- Heavy bleeding during menstruation
- Defects in the uterus or fallopian tubes
- Hypoxia or iron deficiency.

## IMPACT OF ENDOMETRIOSIS

Literature suggests that endometriosis adversely affects the oocytes. It also has a detrimental effect on ovarian quantity which can be determined by anti-Müllerian hormone (AMH). The serum level gets decreased from AMH

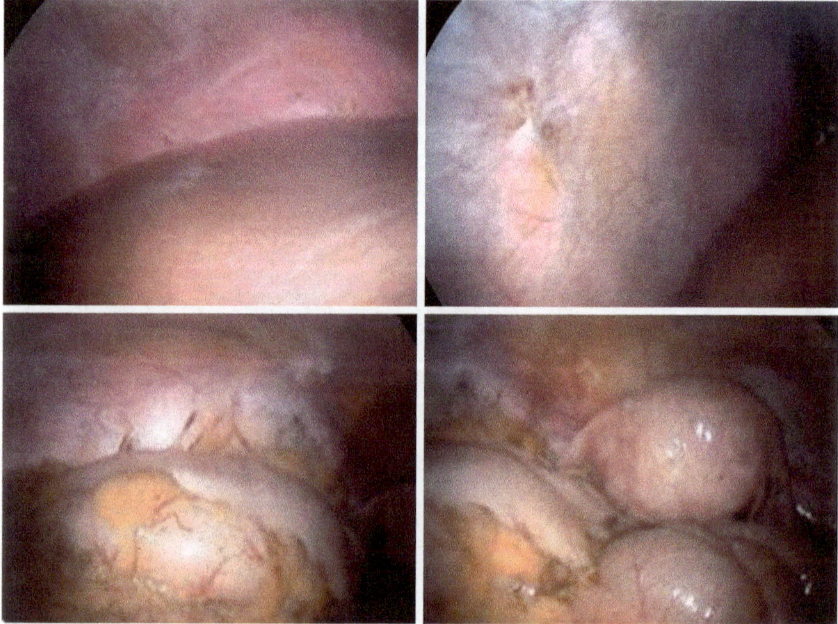

**Fig. 4:** Adhesion observed in endometriosis.
*Source:* Davila GW (2018). What is the pathophysiology of endometriosis?
[online] Available from: https://emedicine.medscape.com/article/271899-overview. [Last accessed March, 2020].

that depicts endometriosis. Surgical excision causes permanent reduction of AMH serum levels.[12]

According to the literature, it is found that quality of life as well as mental health has become poorer among patients suffering from endometriosis with pelvic pain.[13] Women experiencing endometriosis reported various psychological conditions such as anxiety and depression.[14]

In previous studies, neuroendocrine changes were also seen as well as changes such as altered mood and behavior, disorder in sexuality, and appetite. Due to raised stress levels, inflammatory comorbidities such as inflammatory bowel disease, chronic disease, and also autoimmune diseases such as multiple sclerosis and thyroid disease could be seen.[15]

During inflammatory response and scarring, serosa of uterus can also get affected. Severe dyschezia and dyspareunia can be observed as a symptom clinically **(Fig. 4)**.[2]

## CONCLUSION

Though no theory accounts for all, the manifestation of endometriosis but most widely accepted theory of pathogenesis is retrograde menstruation theory. The exact factors for the displacement of the endometrial cells are still unknown. Impaired immunological system is also an important factor responsible for the implantation of endometrial cells outside the uterine cavity.

## REFERENCES

1. Klemmt PAB, Starzinski-Powitz A. Molecular and cellular pathogenesis of endometriosis. Curr Womens Health Rev. 2018;14(2):106-16.
2. Burney RO, Giudice LC. Pathogenesis and pathophysiology of endometriosis. Fertil Steril. 2012;98(3):10.
3. Liu JH (2019). Endometriosis—Gynecology and Obstetrics. [online] Available from: https://www.msdmanuals.com/professional/gynecology-and- obstetrics/endometriosis/endometriosis. [Last accessed March, 2020].
4. Wang Y, Nicholes K, Shih I-M, 2019. The origin and pathogenesis of endometriosis. Annu Rev Pathol. 2020;15:71-95.
5. Goodman LR, Franasiak JM. Efforts to redefine endometriosis prevalence in low-risk patients. BJOG. 2018;125(1):63.
6. Knabben L, Imboden S, Fellmann , Nirgianakis K, Kuhn A, Mueller MD. Urinary tract endometriosis in patients with deep infiltrating endometriosis: prevalence, symptoms, management, and proposal for a new clinical classification. Fertil Steril. 2015;103(1):147-52.
7. Kunz G, Beil D, Huppert P, Noe M, Kissler S, Leyendecker G. Adenomyosis in endometriosis—prevalence and impact on fertility. Evidence from magnetic resonance imaging. Hum Reprod. 2005;20(8):2309-16.
8. Gordts S, Koninckx P, Brosens I. Pathogenesis of deep endometriosis. Fertil Steril. 2017;108(6):872-85.e1.
9. Davila GW, Kapoor D. Endometriosis: Practice Essentials, Background, Pathophysiology. 2019.

10. Vinatier D, Orazi G, Cosson M, Dufour P. Theories of endometriosis. Eur J Obstet Gynecol Reprod Biol. 2001;96(1):21-34.
11. Asghari S, Valizadeh A, Aghebati-Maleki L, Nouri M, Yousefi M. Endometriosis: perspective, lights, and shadows of etiology. Biomed Pharmacother. 2018;106:163-74.
12. Seyhan A, Ata B, Uncu G. The impact of endometriosis and its treatment on ovarian reserve. Semin Reprod Med. 2015;33(6):422-8.
13. Facchin F, Barbara G, Saita E, Mosconi P, Roberto A, Fedele L, et al. Impact of endometriosis on quality of life and mental health: pelvic pain makes the difference. J Psychosom Obstet Gynaecol. 2015;36(4):135-41.
14. La Rosa VL, Barra F, Chiofalo B, Platania A, Di Guardo F, Conway F, et al. An overview on the relationship between endometriosis and infertility: the impact on sexuality and psychological well-being. J Psychosom Obstet Gynaecol. 2019;1-5.
15. Luisi S, Pizzo A, Pinzauti S, Zupi E, Centini G, Lazzeri L, et al. Neuroendocrine and stress-related aspects of endometriosis. Neuro Endocrinol Lett. 2015;36(1):15-23.

# CHAPTER 2

# Diagnosis and Staging of Endometriosis

Anu Agarwal, Sabita Dixit

## INTRODUCTION

Endometriosis is defined as the presence of estrogen-sensitive and endometrial-like tissue outside the uterus, which induces a chronic and inflammatory reaction (Kennedy et al., 2005). While some women with endometriosis experience painful symptoms and/or infertility, others have no symptoms at all.

The exact prevalence of endometriosis is unknown but estimates range from 2% to 10% within the general female population and up to 50% in infertile women (Eskenazi and Warner, 1997; Meuleman et al., 2009).

Apart from the economic burden arising from the women with endometriosis treated in referral centers, endometriosis has a significant effect on various aspects of women's lives including their social and sexual relationship, work, and study (De Graff et al., 2013; Nnoaham et al., 2011; Simoens et al., 2012).

Therefore, there is a significant need to optimize the management of women with endometriosis to improve diagnosis, endometriosis care, and reduce both the personal and social cost of this disease.

Endometriosis diagnosis is based on the women's history, symptom, and signs; the diagnosis is corroborated by physical examination and imaging techniques and finally proven by histology of either a directly biopsied lesion, from a scar, or a tissue collected during laparoscopy.

## ADOLESCENT ENDOMETRIOSIS

Adolescent girls (13–19 years old) constitute around 3–5% of the patients suffering from endometriosis. Most of the girls present with severe dysmenorrhea and school absenteeism, pain interfering with daily activities, not responding to nonsteroidal anti-inflammatory drugs (NSAIDs) and oral contraceptives (OCPs) when taken for pain relief.

## DIAGNOSIS
### Clinical Presentation

Endometriosis should be suspected in women with subfertility, dysmeno-rrhea, dyspareunia, or chronic pelvic pain. However, these symptoms can also be associated with other diseases. Endometriosis may be asymptomatic, even in some women with more advanced disease (ovarian or deeply invasive rectovaginal endometriosis).

## Pain

*Pelvic symptoms:* The pelvic symptoms are cyclical pelvic pain, dysmenorrhea, dysuria, dyspareunia, chronic pelvic pain, cyclical intestinal symptoms like periodic bloating, diarrhea, or constipation (Bellalis et al., 2010; Davis et al., 1993; Luscombe et al., 2009), fatigue/weariness, and infertility.

Adolescents with endometriosis report a high rate of symptoms like— uterine cramping (reported by 100%), cyclical pain (67%), noncyclic pain (39%), constipation or diarrhea (67%), and referred pain (legs and back) by 31% of adolescents with laparoscopically diagnosed endometriosis (Davis et al., 1993).

In women seeking help from general practitioners, the following symptoms were found to be risk factors for endometriosis abdominopelvic pain, dysmenorrhea, heavy menstrual bleeding, infertility, subfertility, dyspareunia, postcoital bleeding, and a previous history of ovarian cyst, irritable bowel syndrome, and pelvic inflammatory diseases.

So, diagnosis of endometriosis should be considered both in gynecological and nongynecological cyclical symptoms (dyschezia, dysuria, hematuria, rectal bleeding, and shoulder pain).

We should be aware of extragenital endometriosis, when bleeding from unusual sites, e.g., epistaxis, cyclical hemopneumothorax, hematochezia, hematuria, umbilical bleeding, and bleeding from previous scars are seen.

## Subfertility and Infertility

When endometriosis is moderate or severe, involving the ovaries and causing adhesions that block tubo-ovarian motility and ovum pickup, it is associated with subfertility.[1]

Although numerous mechanisms (ovulatory dysfunction, luteal insufficiency, luteinized unruptured follicle syndrome, recurrent abortions, altered immunity, and intraperitoneal inflammation) have been proposed,[2] the association between fertility and minimal or mild endometriosis remains controversial.[1,3]

## Spontaneous Abortion

Based on controlled prospective studies, there is no evidence that endometriosis is associated with recurrent pregnancy loss, or that medical or surgical treatment of endometriosis reduces the spontaneous abortion rate.[4-6]

## *Endocrinologic Abnormalities*

Endometriosis has been associated with anovulation, abnormal follicular development with impaired follicle growth, reduced circulating E2 levels during the preovulatory phase, disturbed luteinizing hormone (LH) surge patterns, premenstrual spotting, the luteinized unruptured follicle syndrome, and galactorrhea and hyperprolactinemia.[7]

## *Extrapelvic Endometriosis*

Extrapelvic endometriosis, although often asymptomatic, should be suspected when symptoms of pain or a palpable mass occur outside the pelvis in a cyclic pattern.

## Clinical Examination

Inspection and palpation of abdomen, vulva, vagina, and cervix should be performed for any signs of endometriosis:

- We may find a painful, tender, and hypertrophied episiotomy scar.
- Possible signs of endometriosis include:
  - Uterosacral or cul-de-sac nodularity
  - Painful swelling of the rectovaginal septum
  - Unilateral ovarian cystic enlargement
  - Visible vaginal nodules in the posterior vaginal fornix.

In more advance disease, uterus is often in fixed retroversion and the mobility of the ovaries and fallopian tube is restricted.

Evidence of deeply infiltrative lesion (deeper than 5 mm under the peritoneum) in the cul-de-sac and rectovaginal septum should be sought during menstruation. So, in all women with suspected endometriosis, clinical examination by the way of per abdominal, per speculum, per vaginal, per rectal, and rectovaginal examination, after counseling, should be done. And, we should rule out nonendometriotic causes of pelvic pain.

In adolescent and/or women without previous sexual intercourse, rectal examination can be helpful for the diagnosis of endometriosis.

We should consider diagnosis of endometriosis in women suspected of the disease even if the clinical examination is normal (Chapron et al., 2002).

## Medical Technologies in the Diagnosis of Endometriosis

Diagnosis in adolescents is done through history, physical examination, risk factors and family history combined with imaging studies and biomarkers.

For diagnosing adolescent endometriosis, high level of suspicion should be there.

## Investigations

### Biomarkers

- Apart from research settings, biomarkers are not recommended for routine clinical use (FOGSI, Good clinical practice recommendations on endometriosis).
- *Serum CA-125*: Marker found on derivatives of coelomic epithelium and common to most nonmucinous epithelial ovarian carcinomas.[8] Serum CA-125 has been found to be significantly higher in women with moderate or severe endometriosis and normal in women with minimal or mild disease.[9]
- Serum CA-125 may be of value to rule out ovarian malignancies and presence of extensive peritoneal lesions. In some cases, it may be of some value for treatment follow-up.

  (FOGSI: Good clinical practice recommendations on endometriosis).

  Serial Serum CA-125 determinations may be useful to predict the recurrence of endometriosis after therapy.[10,11]

### Imaging Modalities for Diagnosis of Endometriosis

*Transvaginal sonography in the diagnosis of ovarian endometriosis:* Endometriomas are present in up to 44% of women with endometriosis.[12]

Sonographic features vary from simple cyst to complex cyst with internal echoes to solid masses, usually devoid of internal vascularity but show pericystic flow with high resistance.

Ultrasonologic features of endometriosis are:

- Cystic lesions with diffuse low level internal echoes are described as *ground–glass appearance* is characteristic, with 95% of endometriomas having this appearance **(Fig. 1)**.[13-15]
- Endometriomas show posterior acoustic enhancement.

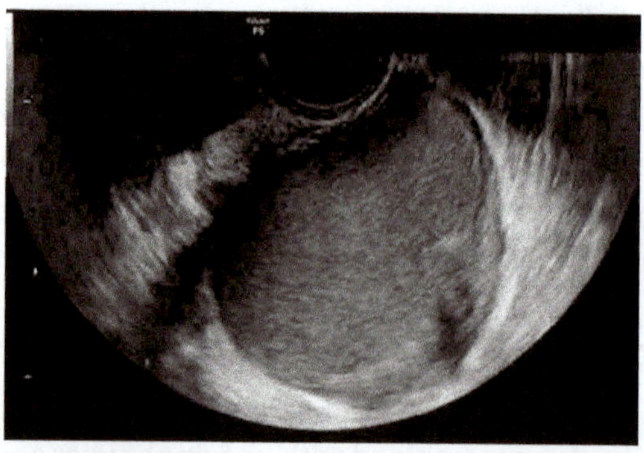

**Fig. 1:** Endometrioma showing classic ground–glass appearance. Note posterior acoustic enhancement, suggesting that this is a cystic lesion rather than a solid lesion.
*Courtesy:* Vansh Fertility and Test Tube Baby Center.

- Multilocularity and echogenic foci in the wall and thick wall have been reported to increase the likelihood that lesion represents an endometrioma.[14]
- Malignant transformations typically clear cell carcinoma and less often endometrioid adenocarcinoma should be suspected in endometriomas that develop solid mural nodules or typically increase in size.[15] Magnetic resonance imaging (MRI) is useful in diagnosing endometriomas suspected of undergoing malignant transformation.
- Sometimes, appearance of endometriomas and hemorrhagic cyst overlaps, and follow-up sonogram, typically in a 6–12-week interval, is suggested. If the lesion is a hemorrhagic cyst, it will resolve or change on follow-up study.

Endometriomas in postmenopausal women may differ in appearance from the typical homogeneous echotexture seen in premenopausal women and may be more heterogeneous with echogenic foci centrally.[16]

A small number of endometriomas may contain a small solid appearing area on ultrasound imaging, and therefore, it can be difficult to distinguish these endometriomas from malignant lesions. [15-17]

Doppler sonographic imaging is suggested, although it may not resolve the diagnosis as the solid area may be due to focal endometrial tissue with internal blood flow, in such cases, additional evaluation with MRI should be considered.

*Transvaginal sonography in the diagnosis of rectal endometriosis:* In women with symptoms and signs of rectal endometriosis, transvaginal sonography is useful for identifying or ruling out rectal endometriosis (Hudelist et al., 2011).

*Three-dimensional (3D) sonography in the diagnosis of rectovaginal endometriosis:* Diagnosis of rectal endometriomas based solely on 3D ultrasound should be limited to highly skilled ultrasound clinicians (Pascual et al., 2010).

*Magnetic resonance imaging:* MRI is not useful to diagnose or exclude peritoneal endometriosis. But, MRI provides a good test to predict whether deep endometriosis has infiltrated the bowel wall and other adjacent organs or not.

## *Laparoscopy in the Diagnosis of Endometriosis*

Laparoscopy with biopsy and histology of suspected lesion is *gold standard* for diagnosis of endometriosis.

However, the quality of both negative and positive laparoscopies depends highly on the abilities of the surgeon performing the laparoscopy.

The experience, skill, and knowledge of the surgeon determine whether endometriosis will be diagnosed, if present. Retroperitoneal and vaginally localized endometriosis can be easily missed, especially if the patient has not been thoroughly examined preoperatively, preferably during anesthesia. A good quality laparoscopy should include systemic checking of:

- The uterus and adnexa
- The peritoneum of ovarian fossae, vesicouterine fold, Douglas, and pararectal spaces
- The rectum and sigmoid
- The appendix and the cecum
- The diaphragm.

Our eyes see what our mind knows. We should have suspicion of these conditions in our mind when we are treating women suffering from endometriosis like:

- Recurrent endometriosis
- Endometriosis and malignancy
- Asymptomatic endometriosis
- Scar endometriosis.

*Recurrent endometriosis:* There are chances for reoccurrence of endometriosis after medical or surgical therapies, because the basic pathophysiology is not corrected.

Treatment is usually symptomatic and removal of the disease as much as possible.

Postoperative recurrence rate is 21% at the end of 2 years and 40–50% at the end of 5 years even in expert hands.[18,19] Risk factors for recurrence are:

- Younger age at the time of surgery[20]
- Bilaterality[19]
- Size of endometriotic lesion
- Revised American Fertility Society (AFS) score > 24[21]
- Preoperative cyst rupture
- Type and extent of surgery.
  (Laparoscopy less risk vs. Laparotomy)
  So, patients should be kept under closed follow-up.

*Endometriosis and malignancy:* Endometriosis is not a malignancy, but it mimics malignancy. It can metastasize to local and distant sites and like malignancy, it can attach, invade, and damage other tissues. Unlike malignancy, it does not result in catabolic state. Incidence of clear cell carcinoma and endometrioid carcinoma are higher among ovarian malignancies associated with endometriosis.[22]

Ovarian cancer is known to develop in 0.3–1.6% of women with endometriosis. There is 4–5-fold increase in ovarian cancer in patients with endometriosis.[23]

A 13-fold increased risk of colorectal cancer in women with adenomyosis with coexistent endometriosis is observed.[23]

*So, women with high-risk factors should be followed closely.*

## ASYMPTOMATIC ENDOMETRIOSIS

Asymptomatic endometriosis means incidental finding of peritoneal, ovarian, or deep endometriosis without pelvic pain or infertility. In asymptomatic patients, diagnosis and treatment become more challenging.

Asymptomatic endometriosis found during laparoscopy or tubal ligation may not warrant any treatment or monitoring. Treatment in the form of excision is not required, since the natural course of the disease is not clear.[24]

In case of incidental finding of endometriosis, it may be removed for tissue diagnosis. We should fully inform and counsel women about any incidental finding of endometriosis.

We should view asymptomatic endometriosis as a marker for potential problems. It does not require treatment but requires monitoring.

The management of symptomatic endometriosis depends upon the relevance of the finding in that particular patient with her particular problem, at that particular time, and the need for therapeutic intervention.

## SCAR ENDOMETRIOSIS

It is a rare disease with nonspecific symptoms like pain and swelling at the scar site especially during menstruation and its incidence is 0.03–0.1%.[25]

The cause for scar endometriosis is often iatrogenic transplantation of endometrial implants (stem cells) to the wound edge during abdominal or pelvic surgeries.

Treating doctor should be aware that cyclical changes of size and intensity of pain noted during menstruation over the scar point toward scar endometriosis.

Hypertrophied and hyperpigmented scars due to hemosiderin deposits are seen; these scars are tender on palpation. Scar endometriosis commonly involves only the skin and the subcutaneous plane and very rarely involves muscle, fascia, and the pelvic organ.[25,26]

### Differential Diagnosis for Scar Endometriosis

The differential diagnoses are stitch granuloma, lipoma, desmoid, tumor, abscess, cyst, keloid, primary or secondary malignant nodules, and inguinal or incisional hernias.

## STAGING OF ENDOMETRIOSIS

Classification of endometriosis has remained challenging in order to provide an effective way to utilize classification in endometriosis-related symptoms (pain, infertility, etc.), treatment plan, prognosis after therapy, recurrence, and association with quality-of-life of women having endometriosis.[1]

Classification should be simple, easy to perform, gives simple description of disease, and correlates well with the problems experienced by women.[27]

There are many staging systems but the most widely used and acceptable is revised American Society for Reproductive Medicine Classification (rASRM). Endometriosis Fertility Index (EFI) has been shown to predict non-IVF pregnancy rates for patients following surgical staging.[27] Women having deep endometriosis should have Enzian[28] classification score, which is a good supplement to rASRM score.

World Endometriosis Society Consensus Statement on Classification of Endometriosis recommends that while better classification system is validated, "all women with endometriosis undergoing surgery should have an rASRM score and stage completed, women with deep endometriosis should have an Enzian classification completed, and women for whom fertility is a future cancer should have an EFI score completed."[29,30]

## American Society for Reproductive Medicine Staging

The revised ASRM staging system is based on appearance, size, and depth of peritoneal and ovarian implants, presence, extent, and type of adnexal adhesions, and degree of obliteration of cul-de-sac.[31]

Morphology of peritoneal and ovarian implants should be categorized as red (red, red pink, and clear lesions), white (white, yellow brown, and peritoneal defects), and black (black and blue lesions) according to color photography provided by ASRM.

Although this staging can assess the extent of endometriosis, but it has intraobserver and interobserver variations.[32,33] This ASRM classification is subjective and correlates poorly with presence of symptoms, pain, and infertility outcomes.[3]

The stages are classified as follows:

- *Stage 1: Minimal (1–5 points)—*
  - Implants are small, few in number, and shallow. Stage 1 does not mean that pain or effect on life is minimal.
- *Stage 2: Mild (6–15 points)—*
  - Implants are more and deeper than superficial implants in stage 1.
- *Stage 3: Moderate (16–40 points)—*
  - There are many deep implants and endometriosis cyst on at least one or both the ovary (chocolate cyst). There may be thin bands (filmy adhesions).
- *Stage 4: Severe (40 or more points)—*
  - There are many deep implants and large cyst on at least one ovary and many dense adhesions throughout the pelvic region.

Endometriosis Foundation of America has divided endometriosis by its anatomical location within pelvic and abdominal cavity and how it affects women because ASRM numerical staging has so many variation and does not give insight into patient pain nor the lesions can be localized:

- *Category 1: Peritoneal endometriosis—*
  - This is the most minimal form in which peritoneum is infiltrated.
- *Category 2: Ovarian endometriomas—*
  - There are endometriomas in ovary, which have the risk of bursting and spreading within pelvic cavity.
- *Category 3: Deep infiltrating endometriosis I (DIE-I)—*
  - It involves organs within pelvic cavity. This can include the ovaries, rectum, uterus, and can even lead to frozen pelvis.
- *Category 4: Deep infiltrating endometriosis II (DIE-II)—*
  - Endometriosis is present within and outside pelvic regions. This can include bowel, appendix, diaphragm, heart, lungs, and even the brain.[34]

Despite of short comings, WES recommends ASRM classification because it is most widely used staging system in practice and research.

It is the rASRM system (partially) incorporated in EFI and Enzian.

## Endometriosis Fertility Index

Endometriosis fertility index is the first validated scoring system that predicts non-IVF pregnancy rates after surgical staging and treatment of endometriosis when the patient has functional gametes and uterus.

Endometriosis fertility index is done on the basis of historical and surgical factors. Historical factors are age, years of infertility, and prior pregnancies.

The surgical factors are total ASRM score, the ASRM endometriosis score, and the least function score, which evaluate functionality of fallopian tubes, fimbriae, and ovaries.

Pregnancy rates decrease significantly in cases of decreased ovarian reserve, older patients, and time span (number of years after surgery).

Endometriosis fertility index does not correlate with pain associated with endometriosis. For non-IVF pregnancy, male and female gametes should be functional. In EFI, uterine abnormality that is significant is not taken into account.

Endometriosis fertility index helps in predicting pregnancy rates over period of 3 years and also helps in deciding treatment option (ART or non-ART).

The time factor in outcome is shown in EFI by flattening of life table curve over time showing decreased PR over time for all EFI score. It has been shown that fecundity is fairly constant after surgery for 12–15 months then it decreases and is generally very low after 2 years **(Table 1)**.

**Table 1:** Endometriosis fertility index:[27] Least function (LF) score.

| Structure | Dysfunction | Description |
|---|---|---|
| *Tube* | | |
| | Mild | Slight injury to serosa of the fallopian tube |
| | Moderate | Moderate injury to serosa or muscularis of the fallopian tube: moderate limitation in mobility |
| | Severe | Fallopian tube fibrosis or mild/moderate salpingitis isthmica nodosa; limitation in mobility |
| | Nonfunctional | Complete tubal obstruction, extensive fibrosis, or salpingitis isthmica nodosa |
| *Fimbria* | | |
| | Mild | Slight injury to fimbria with minimal scarring |
| | Moderate | Moderate injury to fimbria with moderate scarring, moderate loss of fimbrial architecture and minimal intrafimbrial fibrosis |
| | Severe | Severe injury to fimbria, with severe scarring, severe loss of fimbrial architecture and moderate intrafimbrial fibrosis |
| | Nonfunctional | Severe injury to fimbria, with extensive scarring, complete loss of fimbrial |
| *Ovary* | | |
| | Mild | Normal or almost normal ovarian size, minimal or mild injury to ovarian serosa |
| | Moderate | Ovarian size reduced by one-third or more, moderate injury to ovarian surface |
| | Severe | Ovarian size reduced by two-thirds or more; severe injury to ovarian surface |
| | Nonfunctional | Ovary absent or completely encased in adhesions |

*Source*: Adamson GD, Pasta DJ. Endometriosis fertility index: the new, validated endometriosis staging system. Fertil Steril. 2010;94(5):1609-15.

The postoperative least function score is central to the EFI.[28,35] It has predictive power after controlling for the AFS total score and years infertile, although there is some association with AFS scores.[36,37]

## Enzian Classification

In case of deep endometriosis, Enzian staging supplements rASRM staging helping in precise location and extent of deep endometriosis lesions and involvement of retroperitoneal structures or other organs with precise morphology description.

Enzian classification seems to be helpful in planning endometriosis surgery.

Location of deep endometriosis lesions is divided into three compartments. Depth of invasion is rated in three grades:

1. *Grade 1* = Invasion < 1 cm.
2. *Grade 2* = Invasion 1–2 cm; a single lesion is classified only once, i.e., assigned to compartment A, B, or C. When lesion is located on margin between two intersecting compartments, lesion is assigned to large compartment:

    = Rectovaginal septum and vagina

    = Sacrouterine ligament to pelvic wall

    = Rectum and sigmoid colon.
3. *Grade 3* = Invasion > 3 cm.

Deep endometriosis outside the pelvis and invasion of organs is noted separately:

- FA = Adenomyosis
- FB = Bladder
- FU = Intrinsic involvement of ureter
- FI = Intestinal disease cranial to rectosigmoid junction
- FO = Other location such as abdominal endometriosis.

Location used in Enzian classification correlates partly with clinical symptoms and its severity correlates with pain substantially.[28,29]

## REFERENCES


1. American Society for Reproductive Medicine. Revised American Society for Reproductive Medicine Classification of Endometriosis. Am Soc Reprod Med. 1997;5:817-21.
2. Haney AF. Endometriosis-associated infertility. Baillieres Clin Obstet Gynaecol. 1993;7(4):791-812.
3. D'Hooghe TM, Debrock S, Hill JA, Meuleman C. Endometriosis and subfertility: is the relationship resolved? Semin Reporod Med. 2003;21(2):243-54.
4. Matorras R, Rodriguez F, Gutierrez de Teran G, Pijoan JI, Ramón O, Rodríguez-Escudero FJ. Endometriosis and spontaneous abortion rate: a Cohort study in infertile women. Eur J Obstet Gynecol Reprod Biol. 1998;77(1):101-5.
5. Marcoux S, Maheux R Berube S; Canadian Collaborative Group on Endometriosis. Laparoscopic surgery in infertile women with minimal or mild endometriosis. N Eng J Med. 1997;337(4):217-22.
6. Gruppo Italiano per lo stdio dell'Endometriosi. Ablation of lesion or no treatment in minimal mild endometriosis infertile women a randomized trial. Hum Reprod. 1999;14(5):1332-4.
7. Cahill DJ, Hull MGR. Pituitary–ovarian dysfunction and endometriosis. Hum Reprod Update. 2000;6(1):56-66.
8. Bast RC, Klug TL, St-John F, Jenison E, Niloff JM, Lazarus H, et al. A radioimmunoassay using a monoclonal antibody to monitor the course of epithelial ovarian cancer. N Engl J Med. 1983;309(15):883-7.
9. Barbieri RL, Niloff JM, Bast RC Jr, Schactzl E, Kistner RW, Knapp RC. Elevated serum concentrations of CA 125 in patients with advanced endometriosis. Fertil Steril. 1986;45(5):630-4.

10. Adashi EY. Clomiphene citrate-initiated ovulation: a clinical update. Semin Reprod Endocrinol. 1986;4(3):255-76.

11. Ritchie WE. Ultrasound in the evaluation of normal and induced ovulation. Fertil Steril. 1985;43(2):167-81.

12. Busacca M, Vignali M. Ovarian endometriosis from pathogenesis to surgical treatment. Curr Opin Obstet Gynecol. 2003;15(4)321-6.

13. Valentin L. Use of morphology to characterize and manage common adnexal masses. Best Pract Res Clin Obstet Gynaecol. 2004;18(1):71-89.

14. Patel MD, Feldstein VA, Chen DC, Lipson SD, Filly RA. Endometriomas: diagnostic performance of US. Radiology. 1999;210(3):739-45.

15. Taniguchi F, Harada T, Kobayashi H, Hayashi K, Momoeda M, Terakawa N. Clinical characteristics of patients in Japan with ovarian cancer presumably arising from ovarian endometrioma. Gynecol Obstet Invest. 2014;77(2):104-10.

16. Asch E, Levine D. Variations in appearance of endometriomas. J Ultrasound Med. 2007;26(8):993-1002.

17. Alcazar JL, Laparte C, Jurado M, Lopez-Garcia G. The role of transvaginal ultrasonography combined with color velocity imaging and pulsed Doppler in the diagnosis of endometrioma. Fertil Steril. 1997;67(3):487-91.

18. Guo SW. Recurrence of endometriosis and its control. Hum Reprod Update. 2009;15(4):441-61.

19. Selçuk I, Bozdağ G. Recurrence of endometriosis; risk factors, mechanisms and biomarkers; review of the literature. J Turk Ger Gynecol Assoc. 2013;14(2):98-103.

20. Szczepańska M, Skrzypczak J. Risk factors analysis of endometrial cysts recurrence after their surgical removal. Ginekol Pol. 2007;78(11):847-51.

21. Yun BH, Jeon YE, Chon SJ, Park JH, Seo SK, Cho S, et al. The Prognostic Value of Individual Adhesion Scores from the Revised American Fertility Society Classification System for Recurrent Endometriosis. Yonsei Med J. 2015;56(4):1079-86.

22. Yoshikawa H, Jimbo H, Okada S, Matsumoto K, Onda T, Yasugi T, et al. Prevalence of endometriosis in ovarian cancer. Gynecol Obstet Invest. 2000;50(Suppl 1):11-7.

23. Kok VC, Tsai H-J, Su C-F, Lee C-K. The risks for ovarian, endometrial, breast, colorectal, and other cancers in women with newly diagnosed endometriosis or adenomyosis: a population-based study. Int J Gynecol Cancer. 2015;25(6):968-76.

24. Philippine society of reproductive endocrinology and infertility inc. [online] Available from: http://psrei.org/. [Last accessed March, 2020].

25. Wolf GC, Singh KB. Cesarean scar endometriosis: a review. Obstet Gynecol Surv. 1989;44(2):89-95.

26. Chatterjee SK. Scar endometriosis: a clinicopathologic study of 17 cases. Obstet Gynecol. 1980;56(1):81-4.

27. Adamson GD, Pasta DJ. Endometriosis fertility index: the new, validated endometriosis staging system. Fertil Steril. 2010;94(5):1609-15.

28. Keckstein J, Ulrich U, Possover M. ENZIAN klassifikation der tiefinfiltrierenden Endometriose. Zentrallbl Gyankol. 2003;125:291. [online] Available from: http://www.endometriose-sef.de/dateien/ENZIAN_2013_web.pdf. [Last accessed March, 2020].

29. Tuttlies F, Keckstein J, Urich U, Possover M, Schweppe KW, Wustlich M, et al. ENZIAN-score, a classification of deep infiltrating endometriosis. Zentralbl Gynakol. 2005;127(5):275-81.

30. Johnson NP, Hummelshoj L, Adamson GD, Keckstein J, Taylor HS, Abrao MS, et al.; World Endometriosis Society Sao Paulo Consortium. World Endometriosis Society consensus on the classification of endometriosis. Human Repord. 2017;32(2):315-24.

31. The American Fertility Society. Classification of endometriosis. Fertil Steril. 2002;77(6):633-4.

32. Hornstein MD, Gleason RE, Orav J, Haas ST, Friedman AJ, Rein MS, et al. The reproducibility of the revised American Fertility Society classification of endometriosis. Fertil Steril. 1993;59(5):1015-21.
33. Lin SY, Lee RK, Hwu YM, Lin MH. Reproducibility of the revised American Fertility Society classification of endometriosis during laparoscopy or laparotomy. Int J Gynecol Obstet. 1998;60(3):265-9.
34. Hass D, Wurm P, Shamiyeh A, Shebl O, Chvatal R, Oppelt P. Efficacy of the revised Enzian classification: a retrospective analysis. Does the revised Enzian classification solve the problem of duplicate classification in rASRM and Enzian? Arch Gynecol Obstet. 2013;287(5):941-5.
35. Kistner RW, Siegler AM, Behrman SJ. Suggested classification for endometriosis: relationship to interfirtility. Fertil Steril. 1977;28(9):1008-10.
36. Adamson GD, Frison L, Lamb EJ. Endometriosis: studies of a method for the design of a surgical staging system. Fertil Steril. 1982;38(6):659-66.
37. Acosta AA, Buttram VC Jr, Besch PK, Malinak LR, Franklin RR, Vanderheyden JD. A proposed classification of pelvic endometriosis. Obstet Gynecol. 1973;42(1):19-25.

# CHAPTER 3

# Adolescent Endometriosis

*Asha R Rao, Damodar R Rao, M Preethi*

## INTRODUCTION

Endometriosis was frequently described as an enigmatic condition due to many unanswered questions and controversies in its pathogenesis, diagnosis, and management. Endometriosis was once believed to occur in teenagers rarely and was thought to affect women in later reproductive years. With increasing awareness of both healthcare professionals and general population, it is now well-revealed that endometriosis affects significant teenagers.

After introduction of keyhole surgery since 1980s, endometriosis is recognized as a disease that affects adolescent and young women whereas in the beginning, it was believed that it was rare in younger age group.

Endometriosis prevalence in adolescents undergoing keyhole surgery for chronic pelvic pain is reported to be between 19% and 73%. To our surprise, rarely endometriosis has also been notified in premenarcheal girls with some breast development. Diagnosis of adolescent endometriosis is often delayed in the adolescent girls for >6–8 years if high index of suspicion is not there.

Several factors have been described for endometriosis whereas no single theory can explain the cause of symptoms. Genetic factors may seem to play a role whereas lifestyle characteristics and environmental factors also can be related to the development of the disease.

*The rising concern on this topic is because diagnosis of this condition is quite challenging:*

- Existing symptoms of endometriosis in adolescents is persistent chronic pelvic pain, despite medical management like either hormonal contraceptives or pain killers.
- In almost 60–70% of adults with endometriosis, symptoms started even before the women reached 20s.
- These girls tend to have more school absentees during their menses and also take leave more frequently than usual for a longer period of time, despite the use of an oral contraceptive to treat severe primary dysmenorrhea.
- Several symptoms, which are associated with gastrointestinal tract, are seen with these adolescent girls like constipation, diarrhea, nausea, and vomiting.

- Endometriotic lesions are typically clear or red in adolescents and so it is difficult to identify for gynecologists unfamiliar with endometriosis in adolescents and so deeper lesions seem to be rare.
- There is no evidence whether the treatment for adolescent endometriosis may prevent disease progression in their later life.

## RISK FACTORS

Müllerian anomalies most commonly obstructive type is known to be associated with increased risk of endometriosis in teenagers. That may be due to increased retrograde menstruation. Spontaneous resolution of such endometriosis has been reported after surgical correction of obstruction. Similar to adult endometriosis, there is association of family in these young girls as well.[1]

## SYMPTOMS

The major diagnostic symptoms of endometriosis in adolescence are chronic pelvic pain (27–96%) and dysmenorrhea (18–100%). Acyclic pain tends to be more common in these teens than in adults. Other symptoms are urinary symptoms, gastrointestinal symptoms, pelvic mass, irregular menses, dyspareunia, subfertility, migraine, and depression/anxiety. Adolescents should be offered a pain diary in order to document frequency and pain characters.[1,2]

## HISTORY

Past medical history, family history, and physical examination are necessary for evaluation and management of adolescents with a possible endometriosis. Several other pathologies such as appendicitis, pelvic inflammatory disease, bowel disease, Müllerian anomalies or outflow obstruction, musculoskeletal disorders, hernias, and psychosocial complaints should be excluded prior to diagnosing adolescent endometriosis.[2-4]

## EXAMINATION

Inspection of the girl should be done for possible estrogen-dependent body configuration with peripheral fat distribution and also for breast and pubic hair development according to the Tanner system.

A patent outflow tract should be evaluated in these teen adolescents by placing a Q-tip into the vaginal canal. This is very helpful to exclude a possible transverse vaginal septum, vaginal agenesis, or agenesis of the lower vagina. For virgin adolescents, pelvic examination cannot be performed, hence, rectal-abdominal examination is done. Importance should be given for diagnosis of both diffuse and focal pelvic tenderness.[2,5]

## INVESTIGATIONS

Imaging is very helpful in these girls. Ultrasonography and magnetic resonance imaging (MRI) will perform anatomical evaluation, but are not specific for diagnosing endometriosis:

- *Transvaginal ultrasound*: Transvaginal ultrasound is to detect a case of suspected endometriosis even if the pelvic and/or abdominal examination is normal so as to identify endometriomas and deep endometriosis involving the bowel, bladder, or ureter. In case of virgins where a transvaginal scan is not appropriate, consider a transabdominal ultrasound imaging of the pelvis.[6]

- *MRI*: According to some studies, MRI can detect endometrial implants with a sensitivity as high as 60% but due to its high cost, it is better not to use pelvic MRI as the primary investigation to diagnose endometriosis in women with symptoms and signs of endometriosis and consider pelvic MRI only to assess the extent of deep endometriosis involving the bowel, bladder, or ureter.[6]

- *Cancer antigen 125 (CA 125)*: Blood tests, such as CA 125, are very sensitive, but they are not specific, thus is not helpful in the diagnosis of adolescent endometriosis. If a coincidentally reported serum CA 125 level is available, then a raised serum CA 125 (that is 35 IU/mL or more) may be consistent with endometriosis; endometriosis may be present despite a normal serum CA 125 IU/mL.[1,6]

- *Role of diagnostic laparoscopy*: Symptomatic adolescents should be evaluated by *diagnostic laparoscopy* where standard treatment of pelvic pain or dysmenorrhea is not effective. Endometriosis should be staged by using the revised criteria of the American Society for Reproductive Medicine-based classification system. During a diagnostic laparoscopy, it is better to take a biopsy of suspected endometriosis in order to confirm the diagnosis of endometriosis (but be aware that a negative histological result does not exclude endometriosis).[6,7]

Few studies showed that the large numbers of lesions in adolescent populations with endometriosis are red lesions while majority of these lesions were correlated with severe dysmenorrhea and also with complaints of abdominal pain, nausea, constipation, and diarrhea.

Another study had reported peculiar atypical red vascular lesions in 60% of these adolescents teens compared to only 20% of nonadolescents **(Figs. 1A and B)**. Clear lesions are common in adolescent endometriosis but often difficult to visualize and evaluate. Peritoneal defects or windows are manifestations of endometriosis, which are very common in adolescents **(Fig. 2)**.

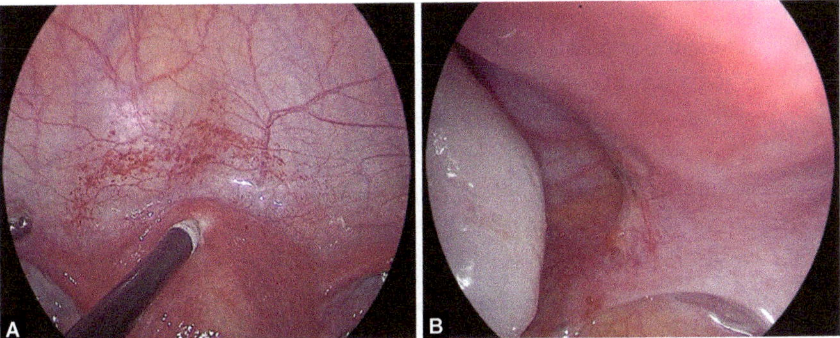

**Figs. 1A and B:** Peculiar atypical red vascular lesions.
*Courtesy:* Rao Hospital.

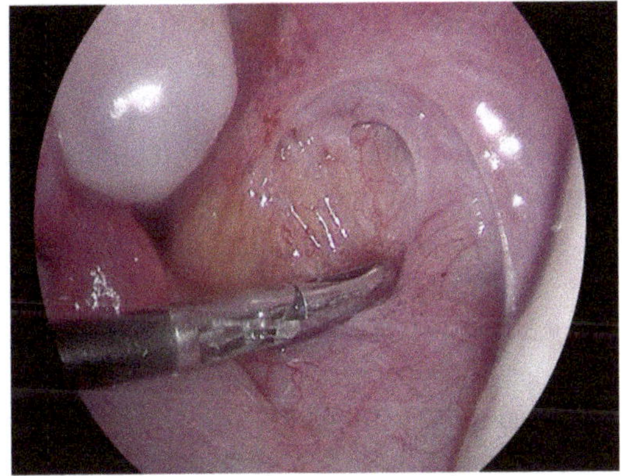

**Fig. 2:** Peritoneal windows in endometriosis.
*Courtesy:* Rao Hospital.

## NATURAL COURSE OF ENDOMETRIOSIS IN TEENAGERS

The natural course of endometriosis in adolescent teens has been always a subject of debate. In adult spontaneous resolution, particularly of superficial lesions have been reported. In teenagers, some authors reported progression of endometriosis lesions in few patients who undergone a second look laparoscopy after ablative therapy of endometriosis. For this reason, some authors are having a belief that teenage endometriosis is a progressive disease.[2,8]

## MEDICAL TREATMENT

- *Nonsteroidal anti-inflammatory drugs (NSAIDs)*: Due to prevalence of severe dysmenorrhea in teenagers, it is better to treat young girls with this symptom with the classical approach of NSAIDs and/or paracetamol.[5,9] Thus, it has to be remembered that both primary dysmenorrhea and endometriosis-associated pain can respond to these kinds of therapies whereas symptomatic improvement does not rule out endometriosis. It is better to communicate this message to both the teenager and her parents/caregivers; with this sort of approach, it is expected that the symptoms will improve and avoid a significant number of further unnecessary investigations including laparoscopy. It is also better to explain that the symptoms of endometriosis may be masked due to NSAIDs, thus allowing the condition to progress further.

- *Hormonal treatment*: Women with suspected or confirmed endometriosis, hormonal treatment may reduce pain, but has no permanent negative effect on subsequent fertility. Thus, it is better to offer hormonal treatment [for example, the combined oral contraceptive (COC) pill or a progestogen] to women with recurrent endometriosis. If the pain is not responding to the COC or NSAIDs treatment, then there is a high likelihood of endometriosis. In this situation, diagnosis of endometriosis with further investigations, including a diagnostic laparoscopy if necessary, would be sensible before using further medical treatment options such as gonadotropin-releasing hormone analogs (GnRHa).

- *Levonorgestrel-releasing intrauterine system (LNG-IUS)*: LNG-IUS can be used successfully for the treatment of endometriosis-associated pain in adults. However, there is a lack of evidence for its use in teenagers. Hence, it may not be appropriate to use LNG-IUS as a first-line empirical treatment for presumed endometriosis in younger teenagers, but this may be an acceptable option for older teenagers, particularly for those who are sexually active.[1,3]

- *Gonadotropin-releasing hormone agonist*: GnRHa treatment is reserved for those teenagers with surgically confirmed disease only. There is, however, concern of overuse of GnRHa in teenagers who are at the critical stage of achieving the peak bone density. Despite this, some authors suggest that GnRHa can be an option for treatment of endometriosis-associated pain in teenagers. There should be a caution in selecting patients for this type of treatment and alternative options, including surgery, should be weighed carefully. GnRHa may be acceptable option for teenagers after the age of 17 years after completion of bone formation.[10]

- *Progestins*: There is a paucity of data on the usage of progestins in teenagers. This is probably because of the long-term use of progestins on bone mineral density (BMD). Data showed that women who used depot medroxyprogesterone acetate (DMPA) on long-term have lower BMD. For this reason, the UK National Institute for Health and Care Excellence (NICE) recommended that care should be taken in recommending DMPA as a contraceptive to adolescents, but that it should be considered only if other methods are not suitable or not acceptable:[6]

- *Dienogest (DNG)*: DNG is a synthetic newer oral progestogen which is highly selective for the progesterone receptor. It has strong progestational effects, moderate antigonadotropic effects, and no androgenic, glucocorticoid, or mineralocorticoid activity.

  *Dienogest* 2 mg once a day can be started at any day of the menstrual cycle and appears to be safe and effective when taken up to 2 years. Current treatments are limited to shorter treatment intervals. DNG is effective in treating symptomatic women with rectovaginal endometriosis even in a particular endometriotic subpopulation of norethindrone acetate (NETA)-"resistant" patients. DNG can be a novel alternative for extragenital endometriosis.

  Treatment of adolescent endometriosis with DNG is not inferior when compared to that with GnRH agonists **(Flowchart 1)**. DNG was found to be successful in those patients with deep infiltrating endometriosis with or without visceral involvement; a slight reduction in BMD is noted only after 24–52 weeks of treatment.[11]

## SURGERY

Surgery is often indicated in those adolescent/teens who have:

- Pain (failed medical management)
- Large endometrioma (>3 cm)[12]
- Moderate or severe disease distorting anatomy
- Infertility.

Surgical options in adolescent teens will include laparoscopy rather than laparotomy. Surgery should be timed ideally in the follicular phase of her menstrual cycle in order to prevent future possibility of recurrences and adhesions. The goal of surgical treatment is the possible removal of visible areas of endometriosis and restores their normal anatomy by adhesiolysis **(Fig. 3)**.[13,14]

The advantages of laparoscopy are:

- Magnification
- Better visualization of subtle lesions
- Less tissue trauma and desiccation
- Smaller incisions
- Speedy postoperative recovery
- Less postoperative adhesions.

Endometriotic lesions are typically clear or red in adolescents and can be difficult to identify for gynecologists unfamiliar with endometriosis in adolescents **(see Figs. 1 and 2)**. Techniques described to enhance visualization of the lesions include moving the laparoscope within millimeters of the

**Flowchart 1:** The American College of Obstetricians and Gynecologists has put forth a stepwise treatment algorithm for treatment of adolescent endometriosis.[2]

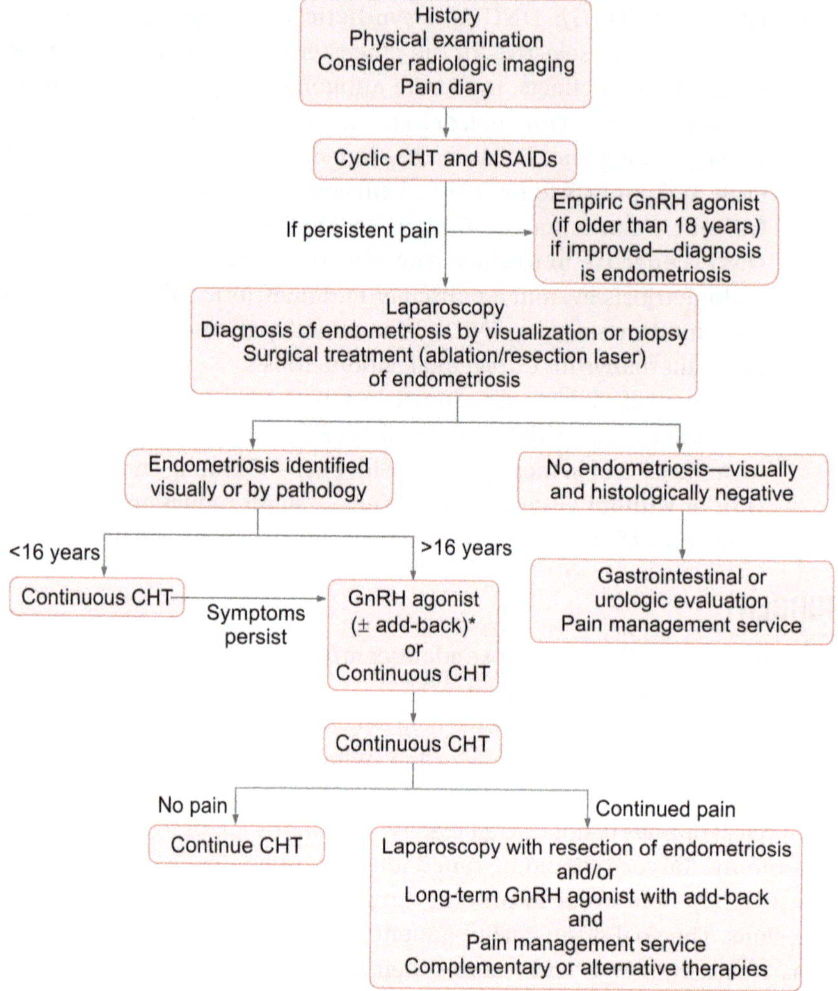


(CHT: combination hormone therapy; GnRH: gonadotropin-releasing hormone; NSAIDs: nonsteroidal anti-inflammatory drugs)
*Add-back indicates use of estrogen and progestin or norethindrone acetate alone.

peritoneum (magnification technique) and filling the pelvis with saline and "diving in" with the laparoscope. Lesions suspicious of endometriosis should be sampled and biopsied and visible lesions should be destroyed, ablated, or excised at the time of initial laparoscopy. Occasionally, biopsy of such inconclusive lesion may not confirm endometriosis and visual diagnosis may suffice so that treatment can be initiated. The American College of Obstetricians and Gynecologists does not recommend "peritoneal stripping" in adolescents based on theoretical concerns (e.g., adhesion formation

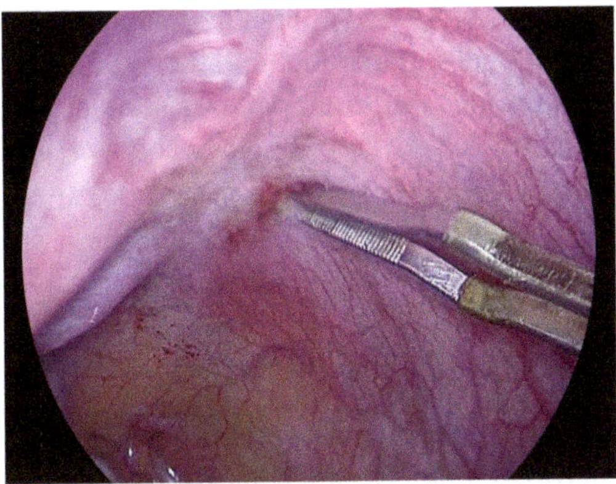

**Fig. 3:** Surface endometriosis electrocoagulation.
*Courtesy:* Rao Hospital.

contributing to bowel obstruction or infertility, or both, and persistent pain). In addition, there is a lack of short-term and long-term outcome data about the procedure.[1,2]

At laparoscopy, most adolescents are diagnosed with early-stage endometriosis (American Society for Reproductive Medicine stage 1 or 2), although there are a number of recent reports of young women presenting with more advanced disease. When counseling families about surgical findings, it is important to communicate that the stage and location of endometriosis is not directly related to the frequency or severity of symptoms. Although typically diagnosed with earlier stage disease, adolescents may still experience substantial pain because the clear and red lesions are more metabolically active and are associated with production of prostaglandin than the "powder burn" lesions which are seen in adult women.

The procedure seems to improve the endometriotic symptoms in 38–100% of adolescents. Laser vaporization and monopolar or bipolar coagulation are the methods used, though no single technique has been shown to be superior than the other. In some studies, it is reported that complete laparoscopic excision by experts can significantly reduce the recurrence rates of endometriosis in adolescents while Yang et al. found a zero rate of recurrence of the disease (diagnosed visually or histologically) after complete laparoscopic excision of the disease in teenagers at a repeat laparoscopy for pain. Even though frequency of adolescents who undergo laparoscopy for persistent recurrent pain is 47.1%, the rate of endometriosis found at surgery was zero.[15]

First-line therapy for adolescents with either surgically diagnosed and destroyed endometriosis or presumed endometriosis includes suppressive hormonal therapy using a continuous combined hormonal contraceptive, a progestin-only agent, 52 µg of LNG-IUS, or DNG. All of these methods have been shown to be effective. Patients may benefit from trying several different types of hormonal suppression until they find their best fit. Because endometriosis is a chronic condition, patients should continue hormonal suppression unless they are actively trying to become pregnant.

Patients who have pain refractory to conservative surgical therapy and suppressive hormonal therapy may often benefit from at least 6 months of GnRH agonist therapy with add-back medicine.

## Endometrial Cysts Management

Endometrioma of ovary is the most common symptomatic presentation of advanced endometriosis in adolescents. Recent publications have reported large number of cases of adolescents with stage III and IV endometriosis. Red lesions are the most usual lesions seen in adolescents with some atypical lesions being common among these teens.[12]

Ovarian endometriomas are usually correlated with more advanced stage of the disease and it is easily understood that these girls will present with more frequent pain. A retrospective study of 63 adolescents with endometrioma found bilateral disease in 22.2% while endometrioma in the right ovary seems to be more frequent than a left endometrioma (65% vs. 57%).[13] In these cases, the preferable surgery is a combined technique of cystectomy and cauterization of the capsule. Interestingly, in a review by Gordts et al., it was found that early ablative surgery can contribute to a lower morbidity, relief of symptoms, and a better quality of life; while another recent published study has reported recurrence rates of endometrioma per patient at 24, 36, 60, and 96 months after laparoscopic cyst enucleation for ovarian endometrioma being 6.4%, 10%, 19.9%, and 30.9%, respectively and all these adolescents had stage III or IV of the disease **(Figs. 4A and B)**.[14]

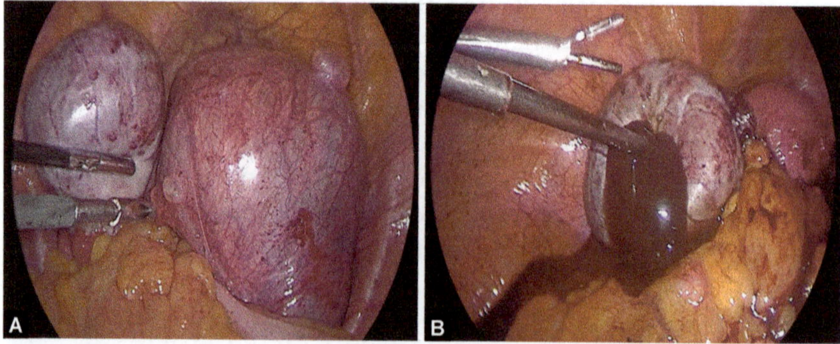

**Figs. 4A and B:** Ovarian endometrioma in a 16-year-old adolescent and drainage of endometriotic cyst.
*Courtesy:* Rao Hospital.

Increasing numbers have been reporting their outcomes following surgical treatment of endometriosis in teenagers. The majority of these publications were included in the aforementioned systematic review by Janssen et al.[10] These publications included treatment either by ablation or excision of endometriosis and some did not specify how endometriosis was treated. Only a few of these articles gave outcome data after surgery.

## ROLE OF POSTOPERATIVE HORMONAL SUPPRESSION

Postoperative hormonal suppression should be offered to adolescents in order to treat symptoms and to prevent disease progression and/or recurrence of the disease while the role of postoperative medical therapy in addition with surgery in improving future fertility of adolescents with endometriosis has not been well-documented.

The recurrence rate of endometriosis in these young women appears to be higher than in older women. In a retrospective cohort study of 57 women, aged ≤21 years, and who were treated initially by excisional surgery, has shown rate of recurrence of symptoms during a follow-up period of 5 years was 56%. The study also showed that the postoperative medical therapy did not influence the recurrence rates.[16]

As reported above, a variety of medical therapies have been used in treating endometriosis during adolescence. Even though further studies are needed, in order to conclude which medical therapy is superior than the other, GnRH agonists seem to be more effective compared with COCs and progestins to prevent disease recurrence. DNG 2 mg is equivalent in efficacy to leuprolide acetate (LA) for reducing endometriosis-associated pelvic pain. DNG is the most effective to reduce the recurrence of endometrioma and therefore the necessity of reoperation for a prolonged period.[11]

*Conjugated equine estrogens as add-back therapy in combination with NETA* will be more effective for increasing total bone mineral content, BMD, and lean mass than using the usual NETA monotherapy. LNG-IUS is accepted for use in the adolescent population for contraception and menorrhagia in sexually active women, but there are not enough data regarding its effectiveness in the treatment of adolescent endometriosis.[17]

In those studies of adults with endometriosis, DNG has shown limited effects on BMD. In a 24-week trial, Strowitzki et al. observed a 0.25% increase in mean lumbar spine BMD with DNG 2 mg versus a decrease of 4.04% with LA.[11]

## RECURRENCE FOLLOWING SURGERY

Tandoi et al.[10] reported high recurrence rates following surgery; during a 5-year follow-up, they found 56% recurrence rate among 57 young women aged ≤21 years. Only 34% of these recurrences were confirmed laparoscopically and in the remaining 66%, the diagnosis of recurrence was based on symptoms or ultrasound findings. By contrast, Yeung et al.[18] found no visual or histological evidence of recurrence in the eight of 17 teenagers (47%) who underwent repeat laparoscopy within 66 months following laparoscopic treatment of endometriosis.

The majority of publications reported use of postoperative medical maintenance treatment such as the COC pill or LNG-IUS. Some groups even advocate the use of GnRHa treatment. As discussed above, LNG-IUS can be inserted at the end of surgery, eliminating the concern of insertion of IUS in the outpatients in this young age patient group.

There is currently no consensus as to whether surgery should be avoided as much as possible or surgical treatment should be considered at an early stage and should also aim to eliminate endometriosis completely. While some recommend a conservative approach due to high recurrence rates, the others suggest early intervention before more severe lesions develop. Further future research may be required to determine which approach would offer a better long-term relief.

## FUTURE TRENDS

Selective estrogen receptor modulators (SERMs) and selective progesterone receptor modulators (SPRMs) are the newer treatment options available for adolescent endometriosis. These drugs act by suppressing estrogen-dependent endometrial growth without any adverse systemic effects like vasomotor symptoms and loss of BMD. Another treatment option is the use of aromatase inhibitors. It is a key enzyme in estrogen biosynthesis and appears to be overexpressed in areas of endometriosis. This drug acts by reducing ovarian as well as local production of estrogens and it can be used in treatment of adolescent endometriosis. Finally, autoimmune modulators may be an effective option of disease treatment with antitumor necrosis factor therapies have been already successfully used to reduce endometriotic growth in animal models, being a promising future treatment model.

## FOLLOW-UP

A careful follow-up of adolescents with history and symptoms of endometriosis is mandatory as it can be a lifelong disease. Patients should be examined every 3–6 months for disease progression. Thus, pain calendar should be monitored while concerns regarding future fertility and quality of life should be enrolled in the diary. Unless contraindicated, most of those patients should be put on COCs after surgery. If the patient does not respond to surgical management or has recurrence of symptoms, other treatment modalities should be considered. A multidisciplinary approach is usually considered including a gynecologist along with surgeon, gastroenterologist, psychologist, and urologist.

## ISSUES OF INTEREST FOR FUTURE CONSIDERATION

Future studies should be ideally focused on the role of early diagnosis of endometriosis and treatment in progression and advancement of the disease process. There is a need to evaluate the course of endometriosis in teenagers as this may likely to improve our understanding for the development of deep endometriosis.

## CONCLUSION

Due to increasing awareness of endometriosis in teenagers, there is increased prevalence of the disease being documented. The clinicians are taking a more proactive approach in the diagnosis and treatment of endometriosis in this teen age group and both medical and surgical treatment options are being better utilized for them. However, a number of unanswered questions and the importance of prospective data collection/international collaboration are mandatory in order to give a better quality of care for these teens.

## REFERENCES

1. ACOG Committee Opinion No. 760: Dysmenorrhea and endometriosis in the adolescent. Obstet Gynecol. 2018;132:e249-58.

2. Deligeoroglou E, Karountzos V, Tsimaris P, Deligeoroglou E. Endometriosis in adolescence: challenges and opportunities for managing future infertility. Int J Gynecol Clin Pract. 2018;5:145.

3. European Society of Human Reproduction and Embryology (ESHRE)(2019). Ovarian stimulation for IVF/ICSI: Guideline of the European Society of Human Reproduction and Embryology. [online] Available from: https://www.eshre.eu/-/media/sitecore-files/Guidelines/COS/ESHRE-COS-guideline_final-09102019_.pdf?la=en&hash=2316EA35F8AFD21C2FB193C33F3BDC272334C901. [Last accessed March, 2020].

4. Taylor HS, Adamson GD, Diamond MP, Goldstein SR, Horne AW, Missmer SA, et al. An evidence-based approach to assessing surgical versus clinical diagnosis of symptomatic endometriosis. Int J Gynaecol Obstet. 2018;142:131-42.

5. Brosens I, Gordts S, Benagiano G. Endometriosis in adolescents is a hidden, progressive and severe disease that deserves attention, not just compassion. Hum Reprod. 2013;28:2026-31.

6. National Institute for Health and Care Excellence (NICE) (2017). Endometriosis: diagnosis and management. [online] Available from: https://www.nice.org.uk/guidance/ng73/resources/endometriosis-diagnosis-and-management-pdf-1837632548293. [Last accessed March, 2020].

7. Miller JA, Missmer SA, Vitonis AF, Sarda V, Laufer MR, DiVasta AD. Prevalence of migraines in adolescents with endometriosis. Fertil Steril. 2018;109:685-90.

8. Benagiano G, Guo SW, Puttemans P, Gordts S, Brosens I. Progress in the diagnosis and management of adolescent endometriosis: an opinion. Reprod Biomed Online. 2018;36:102-14.

9. Kaur KK, Allahbadia G, Singh M. An update on diagnosis and management of adolescent endometriosis—a short communication. Acta Scientific Paediatr. 2019;2:48-50.

10. Tandoi I, Somigliana E, Riparini J, Ronzoni S, Viganó P, Candiani M. High rate of endometriosis recurrence in young women. J Pediatr Adolesc Gynecol. 2011;24:376-9.

11. Ebert AD, Dong L, Merz M, Kirsch B, Francuski M, Böttcher B, et al. Dienogest 2 mg daily in the treatment of adolescents with clinically suspected endometriosis: The VISanne Study to Assess Safety in ADOlescents. J Pediatr Adolesc Gynecol. 2017;30:560-7.

12. Bedaiwy MA, Allaire C, Alfaraj S. Long-term medical management of endometriosis with dienogest and with a gonadotropin-releasing hormone agonist and add-back hormone therapy. Fertil Steril. 2017;107:537-48.

13. Gordts S, Puttemans P, Gordts S, Brosens I. Ovarian endometrioma in the adolescent: a plea for early-stage diagnosis and full surgical treatment. Gynecol Surg. 2015;12:21-30.

14. Vitonis AF, Baer HJ, Hankinson SE, Laufer MR, Missmer SA. A prospective study of body size during childhood and early adulthood and the incidence of endometriosis. Hum Reprod. 2010;25:1325-34.

15. Yang Y, Wang Y, Yang J, Wang S, Lang J. Adolescent endometriosis in China: a retrospective analysis of 63 cases. J Pediatr Adolesc Gynecol. 2012;25:295-9.

16. Sadler Gallagher J, Feldman HA, Stokes NA, Laufer MR, Hornstein MD, Gordon CM, et al. The effects of gonadotropin-releasing hormone agonist combined with add-back therapy on quality of life for adolescents with endometriosis: a randomized controlled trial. J Pediatr Adolesc Gynecol. 2017;30:215-22.

17. Özyer S, Uzunlar Ö, Özcan N, Yeşilyurt H, Karayalçin R, Sargin A, et al. Endometriomas in adolescents and young women. J Pediatr Adolesc Gynecol. 2013;26:176-9.

18. Yeung P, Sinervo K, Winer W, Albee RB. Complete laparoscopic excision of endometriosis in teenagers: is postoperative hormonal suppression necessary? Fertil Steril. 2011;95:1909-12.

# CHAPTER 4

# Management of Pain in Endometriosis

*Rajeev Agarwal, Kriti Agarwal, Apoorva Pallam Reddy*

## INTRODUCTION

Endometriosis is a common benign gynecological condition defined by the presence of endometrial glands and stroma in sites outside the uterus such as ovaries, rectovaginal septum, pelvis, etc. with a highly variable clinical and surgical picture. Its etiopathogenesis remains elusive and there appears to be a polygenic and multifactorial pattern of inheritance. Endometriosis affects 6–10% of women of reproductive age[1] with prevalence rate as high as greater than one-third of women with infertility and two-thirds of women with chronic pelvic pain.[2] Endometriosis is frequently associated with dysmenorrhea, chronic pelvic pain, deep dyspareunia, dyschezia, and infertility. Ballard et al. found that 83% of women with endometriosis reported one or more of these symptoms to their general practitioners when compared with just 29% of controls.[3] Pain symptoms increase as depth of lesion increases, but no correlation has been found between pain intensity and stage of disease and progression can be highly unpredictable.

## PATHOPHYSIOLOGY

Activated macrophages release cytokines, growth factors, and prostaglandins during menstruation in women who do not have endometriosis in order to regulate the peritoneal cavity by removing red blood cells, tissue fragments, and foreign endometrial cells. Women with endometriosis have a higher level of activated peritoneal macrophages. Therefore, the increased expression of cytokines and growth factors from the macrophages and their effects on the peritoneal environment is associated with the pathophysiology of endometriosis The cause of endometriosis-associated pain is unknown, but it has been suggested that peritoneal inflammation involving growth factors and cytokine production by activated macrophages, adhesion formation and irritation or direct invasion of pelvic floor nerves by infiltrating endometriotic implants may be responsible **(Box 1)**.[4]

Three well-recognized forms of endometriosis have been described here:[5]

1. *Peritoneal endometriosis* corresponds to minimal or mild endometriosis and usually no progression is observed.

> **Box 1:** Mechanisms of pain in endometriosis.
> - Distortion of pelvic anatomy
> - Pelvic adhesions
> - Cyclical bleeding within endometrial lesions
> - Inflammation in peritoneal cavity and fluid
> - Irritation and infiltration of nerves
> - Neurogenesis
> - Neuropathic hyperalgesia

2. *Ovarian endometriosis* is characterized by superficial ovarian implants or endometriotic cysts which may be adherent to the posterior aspects of the broad ligament.

3. *Deep infiltrating endometriosis (DIE)* involving the bowel, bladder, and rectovaginal septum is often associated with pelvic adhesions.

## CLINICAL FEATURES

Despite the increasing awareness of endometriosis, there are often significant delays between the onset of symptoms to definitive diagnosis, with a mean latency of 8 years in the UK and 11.7 years in the USA.[6] One reason for this delay is the significant overlap in symptoms with other conditions such as pelvic inflammatory disease, irritable bowel syndrome, urinary tract infection, interstitial cystitis, and depression. Another reason can be that women may delay seeking medical attention in the misconception that painful symptoms are part of a "normal" menstruation. However, it is quintessential to be aware of classical symptoms of endometriosis, to pick it up before much of damage has been done. The diagnosis of endometriosis is first suspected based on the history, then investigated by physical examination and imaging.

Endometriosis afflicts women of reproductive age; the average age at first diagnosis is 28 years. Endometriosis is frequently associated with dysmenorrhea, chronic pelvic pain, deep dyspareunia, dyschezia, and infertility. Dysmenorrhea is typically defined as triple dysmenorrhea, that is, it begins before onset of menstrual cycles, continues throughout, and persists after cessation of periods. Additionally, it is progressive in nature and tends to get worse with successive cycles due to the subsequent scarring with each monthly bleed. Endometriosis should be considered especially if patients present with dysmenorrhea after having previous pain-free menstrual cycles. Dyschezia during menstruation and deep dyspareunia are stronger predictors of DIE (74.5% sensitivity, 68.7% specificity, 2.4 positive likelihood ratio, and 0.4 negative likelihood ratio).[7]

Mathias et al. underlined also that women diagnosed with endometriosis reported maximum health distress, pain during or after intercourse, and interference with activities because of pain.[8] In addition, women with endometriosis often experience higher incidents of depression and emotional distress due to the uncertainty of diagnosis, unpredictability of symptoms and repeated dismissal of their experiences.

Routine vaginal examination alone is insufficient to make a diagnosis of endometriosis. However, the location and extent of endometriosis can sometimes be determined by clinical examination, especially endometriomas can be palpated through the fornices and tender nodularity in pouch of Douglas (POD) is suggestive of DIE. Particular emphasis should be placed on the visualization of lesions which appear as dark-blue nodules in posterior fornix and increase in size during menstruation.

## DIAGNOSIS

Recent advances in imaging modalities, including transvaginal ultrasound and magnetic resonance imaging, have improved the noninvasive preoperative diagnosis of endometriosis. Transvaginal ultrasonography can be used to identify size and location of endometriotic cysts and bladder lesions, but it may be difficult to distinguish among ovarian endometriomas, cysts, tumors, ectopic pregnancies, tubal cysts or abscesses. Endorectal ultrasonography is a reliable tool but is limited to identifying rectal infiltration associated with deep pelvic endometriosis. MRI can be used to detect up to 82% of endometriomas $\geq 1$ cm and 50% of hemorrhagic lesions $\leq 5$ mm due to the small implant size and variable appearance.[9]

Diagnostic laparoscopy for visualization and biopsy of lesions remains the gold standard for diagnosis after ruling out other causes of pelvic pain, such as upper genital tract infection, adenomyosis, and pelvic inflammatory disease. It is important to note that not all endometriosis lesions are visualized at surgery; lesions may be hidden by pelvic organs or adhesions. Therefore, techniques such as peritoneal fluid aspiration, adhesiolysis, and mobilization of adherent structures such as ovaries from the pelvic wall and biopsy of lesions are typically performed to thoroughly examine the cul-de-sac and pelvic organs and confirm the presence of endometriosis.

## MEDICAL TREATMENT

### Analgesics

Nonsteroidal anti-inflammatory drugs (NSAIDs) are widely used as a first-line treatment of endometriosis-associated pain. Elevated prostaglandin levels in the peritoneal fluid and endometriotic tissue of women with endometriosis support their use. A Cochrane review on the role of NSAIDs in treating endometriosis-related pain analyzed one randomized controlled trial (RCT) comparing naproxen sodium (275 mg, four times daily) with placebo but found no significant difference.[9,10] No evidence shows whether any individual

NSAID is more effective than another. Another study that investigated the use of a cyclo-oxygenase-2 inhibitor (rofecoxib) against a placebo (n = 28) reported significant improvement of dysmenorrhea, dyspareunia and chronic pelvic pain.[11] Although that study reported no adverse effects, Merck & Co. has since withdrawn rofecoxib because of its cardiovascular toxicity.[12]

There are no other RCTs on the use of analgesics (paracetamol, aspirin, ibuprofen, opioids) for treating endometriosis-associated pain.[13]

Specialist help from a multidisciplinary pain team may be required for complex cases, where pain-modulating drugs such as pregabalin or gabapentin may be considered, or low-dose amitriptyline.[14]

> *Category:* NSAIDs
> *Mechanism of action:* Reversible inhibition of COX-1 and COX-2 enzymes
> *Dose:* Ibuprofen—400 mg q4 6 hourly, naproxen—500 mg q1 2 hourly

## Hormonal Therapies for Treating Endometriosis-related Pain

Endometriosis is a progressive disease which gets exacerbated with each monthly bleed due to the increasing collection of menstrual blood in pelvis due to retrograde menstruation, leading to adhesions. Thus, hormonal suppression to achieve amenorrhea is considered a medical approach for treating the disease and its symptoms. Currently, combined oral contraceptive pills (COCPs), progestogens, antiprogestogens, gonadotropin-releasing hormone (GnRH) agonists, antagonists, and aromatase inhibitors (AIs) are in clinical use. The European Society of Human Reproduction and Embryology (ESHRE) guideline states that it is reasonable to commence empirical treatment with analgesia and/or hormones before a diagnosis of endometriosis is confirmed, provided woman has been counseled thoroughly about the efficacy, adverse effect profile, and availability of the different management options.[13]

### Combined Hormonal Contraception

Modern low-dose COCP is now widely used to treat endometriosis-related pain as it offers many practical advantages, including contraceptive protection and cycle control apart from alleviating symptoms in 74% of cases. A recent double-blind, randomized, placebo-controlled trial studied the effectiveness of low-dose COCP compared with placebo for endometriosis-associated pain over four cycles, and concluded that pain scores for the COCP group were significantly reduced compared with placebo.[15]

Changing from cyclical to continuous treatment may improve symptoms; however, moderate-to-severe adverse effects such as irregular bleeding, weight gain, headache, thrombophlebitis, pulmonary embolism, cerebral thrombosis and hemorrhage, hypertension, benign liver tumors, and gallbladder disease have been reported in 14% of women.[16]

Category: Combined hormonal contraceptive (ethinyl estradiol with norethindrone, norgestrel, levonorgestrel or desogestrel)
Mechanism of action: Inhibit FSH and LH, enhanced apoptosis of endometrial implants, decrease cell proliferation
Dose: Continuously or cyclical for 3 months or more
Route:
1. Oral-20 µg ethinylestradiol, 150 µg desogestrel
2. Ring-3-weekly vaginal rings (15 µg of ethinylestradiol and 120 µg etonogestrel)
3. Patch-weekly transdermal (60 µg of ethinylestradiol and 6 mg of 17-deacetylnorgestimate)

## Progestogens and Antiprogestogens

The ESHRE recommends that clinicians take the different side effect profiles of progestagens and antiprogestagens into account when prescribing these drugs, especially irreversible side effects (e.g., thrombosis, androgenic side effects).[13] There was no evidence of a benefit with depot or oral progestogens over other treatments (COCP or leuprolide acetate) for endometriosis-related symptoms.[17]

A recent Cochrane review concluded that medroxyprogesterone acetate (100 mg daily) is significantly more effective in reducing all symptoms when compared with placebo; however, its use was associated with significantly more cases of acne and edema.

No studies have assessed the effectiveness of the progestogen-only pill Cerazetteâ for endometriosis, and the recommendation to offer It is a pragmatic approach based on better side effect profile compared to combined oral contraceptive (COC).

The levonorgestrel-releasing intrauterine system (LNG-IUS) releases levonorgestrel directly into the uterine cavity at a relatively constant rate of 20 µg/day for 5 years. Levonorgestrel exerts strong local activity rendering the endometrium atrophic and inactive, although ovulation is usually not suppressed. RCTs on LNG-IUS have shown that it significantly improves endometriosis-related pain, but this was not significantly different when compared with the effect of leuprolide acetate, aGnRH agonist.[17,18] However, LNG-IUS has a significantly better adverse effects profile as the action is local rather than systemic.[19]

Dienogest is a newer progestogen-only hormone preparation for the treatment of endometriosis. Daily dienogest 2 mg significantly reduces the severity of endometriosis and dyspareunia and is comparable to GnRH agonists.

Dienogest is contraindicated in undiagnosed vaginal bleeding and during pregnancy and lactation, active thromboembolic disorder or a history of cardiovascular disease, diabetes and severe hepatic disease, a history of liver tumors or sex hormone-dependent malignancies. If cholestatic jaundice or pruritis develops, dienogest should be stopped. Although ovulation is inhibited in most patients, dienogest is not a contraceptive and use of a nonhormonal method is recommended while taking dienogest. The menstrual cycle resumes within 2 months of stopping the drug.

*Anti-progestogens* (i.e., a substance that prevents cells from making or using progesterone) such as gestrinone exert antiproliferative effects on the endometrium while maintaining serum estradiol levels in the early to mid-follicular phase, thereby having a better adverse effect profile by avoiding the bone mass loss and hypoestrogenism associated with the use of progestogen-only.[17]

Both continuous progestagens and continuous gestrinone are effective therapies for the treatment of painful symptoms associated with endometriosis.[13]

---

*Category:* Progestin-only preparations
*Mechanism of action:* Inhibit follicle-stimulating hormone (FSH) and luteinizing hormone (LH), enhanced apoptosis of endometrial implants, decrease cell proliferation
*Dose:*
- Norethindrone—2.5 mg/day up to 30 mg/day orally
- Medroxyprogesterone—10 mg/day up to 50 mg/day orally or as depot of 150 mg IM every 3 months
- Cyproterone acetate—12.5 mg/day orally
- Levonorgestrel IUS—52 mg releasing 20 µg/day for 5 years
- Dienogest—2 mg daily orally

---

*Category:* Antiprogestin
*Mechanism of action:* Prevents cells from making or using progesterone, exert anti-proliferative effects on the endometrium
*Dose:* Gestrinone orally 2.5 mg weekly

---

## Gonadotropin-releasing Hormone Agonists

Gonadotropin-releasing hormone agonists (nafarelin, leuprolide, buserelin, goserelin, or triptorelin), deplete the pituitary of endogenous gonadotropins and inhibit further synthesis, thus inducing a hypoestrogenic state resulting in the interruption of the menstrual cycle, and endometrial atrophy and amenorrhea. A Cochrane review of 41 RCTs concluded that GnRH agonists were more effective than placebo but were inferior to LNG-IUS or danazol for relieving endometriosis-associated pain, given its worse adverse effects profile. The hypoestrogenic effects of GnRH agonists include loss of bone mass of up to 13% at 6 months (reversible with discontinuation of therapy), therefore, the simultaneous use of hormonal add-back therapy is recommended. Hormonal add-back therapy has not been shown to reduce the efficacy of GnRH agonists. This can be explained by the estrogen threshold theory, which suggests that lower levels are needed to protect bone and cognitive function and to avoid/minimize menopausal symptoms such as hot flushes, sleep disturbance, and mood swings than to activate endometriotic tissue.[20-23] Although evidence is limited regarding dosage or duration of treatment, nonetheless special consideration to be given to GnRH agonists in young women and adolescents, since these women may not have reached maximum bone density.

> *Category:* GnRH agonists
> *Mechanism of action:* Chronic administration results in decreased follicle-stimulating hormone (FSH) and luteinizing hormone (LH) resulting in decreased steroid synthesis
> *Dose:* Leuprolide—3.75 mg monthly or 11.25 mg/3 monthly IM, with add-back therapy of norethindrone 5 mg/day

## Gonadotropin-releasing Hormone Antagonist

Designing an effective oral GnRH antagonists has been a major drug development goal for the treatment of endometriosis-associated pain. The difficulty has been finding a potent drug that simultaneously blunts hypoestrogenic side effects. A first-generation nonpeptide GnRH antagonist, NBI-42902 was developed and described in 2005, but subsequent human studies showed inhibition of the liver P450 enzymes. Elagolix, a second-generation GnRH antagonist, was subsequently developed with rapid onset of action, good tolerability, and no changes in hepatic enzymes. In addition, its therapeutic and hypoestrogenic effects are rapidly reversed after cessation of therapy. Furthermore, there is a dose-dependent decrease in dysmenorrhea and nonmenstrual pelvic pain in women with endometriosis. Additionally, elagolix is clinically efficacious at two doses (200 or 150 mg daily), allowing the drug to be tailored according to individual needs. Other advantages of elagolix include its immediate suppression of pituitary gonadotrophs, avoiding the initial 1–2 week flare-up effect of GnRH agonists and thereby providing immediate therapeutic effect.

## Aromatase Inhibitors

Aromatase inhibitors have been studied for treating endometriosis despite the controversies surrounding the evidence for increased expression of aromatase P450 in endometriotic tissue.[24] The most common third-generation AIs letrozole and anastrozole are reversible AIs, competing with androgens for aromatase-binding sites. The adverse effects are mostly hypoestrogenic and include vaginal dryness, hot flushes, and diminished bone mineral density. Earlier reports of increased cardiovascular risks have not been substantiated.[13]

A systematic review found that treatment with oral letrozole plus norethisterone acetate (NEA) or desogestrel, or anastrozole as vaginal suppository (250 µg daily) or orally (1 mg daily) in combination with oral contraceptive pill (OCP) resulted in a significant decrease of endometriosis-associated pain in premenopausal women. The same appears to be true for letrozole plus either NEA or triptorelin, although letrozole plus triptorelin resulted in more side effects than NEA. The authors concluded that in women with pain from rectovaginal endometriosis refractory to other medical or surgical treatment, clinicians can consider prescribing AIs in combination with OCPs, progestagens, or GnRH analogs, as they reduce endometriosis-associated pain.[24]

> *Category:* Aromatase inhibitors
> *Mechanism of action:* Blocks conversion of androgen to estrogen decreasing growth of ectopic implants
> *Dose:* Letrozole-2.5 mg/day, anastrozole-1 mg/day

## SURGICAL TREATMENT

The ESHRE supports a "see and treat" approach, but acknowledges that symptoms do not always relate to the severity of clinical disease, and unexpected severe disease may be discovered at initial laparoscopy, which may require further counseling and subsequent surgical treatment. Also, laparoscopy that reveals minimal or mild endometriosis may be difficult to interpret, as the findings may be nonspecific and not necessarily the cause of pain, and if treated at laparoscopy, might not be successful in treating the pain. It is important to note that the response to hormonal therapy has not been shown to always predict the presence or absence of endometriosis.

A woman with endometriosis should receive appropriate preoperative counseling including increased risk of bowel and bladder in DIE, injury to ureters in severely adherent endometrioma, recurrence of pain symptoms and fertility issues. A minimally invasive approach provides superior views of the pelvic organs and is associated with less pain, shorter hospital stay, quicker recovery, and better cosmesis. Laparotomy may rarely be necessary for advanced disease with extensive adhesions or when there is adjoining organ involvement. Nonetheless, both are equally effective. Surgical procedures include excision, fulguration or laser ablation of peritoneal endometriotic implants; excision, drainage, or ablation of endometriomas; resection of rectovaginal nodules; and adhesiolysis.

### Surgery for Endometrioma-associated Pain

Laparoscopic excision of ovarian endometriotic cyst walls (≥3 cm) is superior to drainage and coagulation by bipolar diathermy for treating the recurrence of dysmenorrhea, dyspareunia and nonmenstrual pain as well as reducing the rates of subsequent surgery.[25] While the superiority of excision over drainage and coagulation/ablation might be expected, concerns about excessive resection of ovarian tissue compromising future fertility remain, with a reported risk of ovarian failure after bilateral ovarian endometrioma cystectomy of 2.4%.[26] It should be noted that endometriomas are strongly associated with DIE.[27] Clinicians can use oxidized regenerated cellulose during operative laparoscopy for endometriosis, as it prevents adhesion formation. Additionally, ovarian suspension to abdominal wall following cystectomy may prevent POD obliteration with subsequent monthly bleeds. Postoperative hormonal therapy may not improve the outcome of surgery but is an important adjunct to surgery to prolong the symptom-free interval and prevent recurrence of symptoms. Moreover, as there is no proven harm, so postoperative hormonal therapy could be prescribed for other indications, such as contraception or secondary prevention.[13]

In women operated for endometriosis, clinicians are recommended to prescribe postoperative use of a LNG-IUS or a combined hormonal contraceptive for at least 18–24 months, as one of the options for the secondary prevention of endometriosis-associated dysmenorrhea, but not for nonmenstrual pelvic pain or dyspareunia.[13]

## Surgery for Deep Infiltrating Endometriosis-associated Pain

Deep infiltrating endometriotic nodules may involve the uterosacral ligaments, pelvic side walls, rectovaginal septum, vagina, bowel, bladder, or ureter. Bowel endometriosis usually affects the rectosigmoid colon and can be associated with symptoms such as bowel cramping, diarrhea, or dyschezia.[28]

Medical management of DIE with colorectal extension is usually suppressive and not curative and is often associated with significant adverse effects.[29] It is unclear whether medical management prevents disease progression; however, discontinuing medical treatment commonly results in the recurrence of symptoms.[30]

It is widely agreed that severe endometriosis, especially in symptomatic DIE with colorectal extension, requires surgical treatment. Surgical strategies include superficial shaving, discoid resection or segmental resection of the involved bowel segments to remove the endometriotic nodules. Although there is an ongoing debate about the indication for shaving nodules as opposed to segmental resection, most studies have reported improvement in pain outcome, quality-of-life and gynecological and digestive symptoms after surgery for colorectal endometriosis. The reported intraoperative complication rate was 2.1%, and the total postoperative complication rate was 13.9% (9.5% minor, 4.6% major).[31] The recurrence rates following colorectal endometriosis surgery in studies with more than 2 years of follow-up were 5–25%.[28]

Surgical treatment for bladder endometriosis is usually excision of the lesion and primary closure of the bladder wall. Ureteral lesions may be excised after stenting the ureter; however, segmental excision with end-to-end anastomosis or reimplantation may be necessary if there are intrinsic lesions or significant obstruction.[14]

## Hysterectomy for Endometriosis

Hysterectomy with bilateral salpingo-oophorectomy is generally reserved for women with debilitating symptoms attributable to endometriosis who have completed childbearing and in whom other medical therapies have failed. There are no RCTs on hysterectomy (with or without oophorectomy) for treating endometriosis-associated pain, but a review concluded that hysterectomy was successful in many women, but not all.[32]

An informed consent should be taken in this context from all patients. The success of this approach is attributed to debulking of the disease and the resulting surgical menopause causing endometrial tissue atrophy. Ovarian conservation at hysterectomy presents a sixfold greater risk for the development of recurrent pain and an 8.1 times greater risk of reoperation. Hysterectomy is also used successfully to treat idiopathic dysmenorrhea and adenomyosis.[33] The 2014 ESHRE guidelines suggest combined estrogen and progestogen therapy or tibolone for treating menopausal symptoms in women with surgically induced menopause because of endometriosis, at least up to the age of natural menopause.[13]

## Nerve Interrupting Surgeries

An alternative strategy for controlling endometriosis-related pain is interrupting the nerve pathways. A 2005 Cochrane review concluded that laparoscopic uterosacral nerve ablation conferred no additional benefit over conservative surgery, while presacral neurectomy combined with laparoscopic ablation of endometriotic tissue significantly improved dysmenorrhea and reduced severe midline pain at 6 and 12 months. However, performing presacral neurectomy requires a high degree of skill and is associated with increased risk of adverse effects such as bleeding, constipation, painless first stage of labor, urinary urgency, and is seldom performed.[34]

## ADJUNCT THERAPY

An RCT investigating the use of nutritional supplements on endometriosis demonstrated that 2-month high-dose vitamin E and C therapy was associated with significant improvement in pain.[35] It has been suggested that there is an inverse association between body mass index and endometriosis. This association may correlate with lower peripheral body fat distribution and with less estrogen resistance.[14]

A small Italian study in 2014 suggested that some mood or anxiety disorders, high alexithymia, and malfunctioning obsessive-compulsive symptoms are more frequent in women with endometriosis than in the general population.[36] Thus, some women with endometriosis may benefit from working with a counselor/psychologist to develop strategies on breaking the pain cycle, dealing with stress and anxiety and resolving personal negative feelings.[14]

## KEY CONTENT

- The nonspecific signs and symptoms of endometriosis contribute to significant diagnostic delay.
- Treatment for endometriosis-related pain symptoms includes a range of medical and surgical options.
- Minimally invasive surgery should be performed by a surgeon trained to undertake surgical treatment for mild to moderate disease, thereby avoiding the need for repeat laparoscopy in the absence of severe disease, i.e., a "see and treat" policy.

## REFERENCES


1. Eskenazi B, Warner ML. Epidemiology of endometriosis. Obstet Gynecol Clin North Am. 1997;24(2):235-58.
2. Practice bulletin no. 114: management of endometriosis. Obstet Gynecol. 2010;116(1):223-36.
3. Ballard KD, Seaman HE, de Vries CS, Wright JT. Can symptomatology help in the diagnosis of endometriosis? Findings from a national case-control study–Part 1. BJOG. 2008;115(11):1382-91.
4. Berkley KJ, Rapkin AJ, Papka RE. The pains of endometriosis. Science. 2005;308(5728):1587-9.
5. Nisolle M, Donnez J. Peritoneal endometriosis, ovarian endometriosis, and adenomyotic nodules of the rectovaginal septum are three different entities. Fertil Steril. 1997;68(4):585-96.
6. Husby GK, Haugen RS, Moen MH. Diagnostic delay in women with pain and endometriosis. Acta Obstet Gynecol Scand. 2003;82(7):649-53.
7. Chapron C, Barakat H, Fritel X, Dubuisson JB, Bréart G, FauconnierA. Presurgical diagnosis of posterior deep infiltrating endometriosis based on a standardized questionnaire. Hum Reprod. 2005;20(2):507-13.
8. Mathias SD, Kuppermann M, Liberman RF, Lipschutz RC, Steege JF. Chronic pelvic pain: prevalence, health-related quality of life, and economic correlates. Obstet Gynecol. 1996;87(3):321-7.
9. Brosens I, Puttemans P, Campo R, Gordts S, Kinkel K. Diagnosis of endometriosis: pelvic endoscopy and imaging techniques. Best Pract Res Clin Obstet Gynaecol. 2004;18(2):285-303.
10. Allen C, Hopewell S, Prentice A, Gregory D. Nonsteroidal anti-inflammatory drugs for pain in women with endometriosis. Cochrane Database Syst Rev. 2009;(2):CD004753.
11. Kauppila A, Ronnberg L. Naproxen sodium in dysmenorrhea secondary to endometriosis. Obstet Gynecol. 1985;65(3):379-83.
12. Cobellis L, Razzi S, De Simone S, Sartini A, Fava A, Danero S, et al. The treatment with a COX-2 specific inhibitor is effective in the management of pain related to endometriosis. Eur J Obstet Gynaecol Reprod Biol. 2004;116(1):100-2.

13. Dunselman GA, Vermeulen N, Becker C, Calhaz-Jorge C, D'Hooghe T, De Bie B, et al. ESHRE guideline: management of women with endometriosis. Hum Reprod. 2014;29(3):400-12.

14. Hoo WL, Hardcastle R, Louden K. Management of endometriosis-related pelvic pain. Obstet Gynaecol. 2017;19(2):131-8.

15. Harada T, Momoeda M, Taketani Y, Hoshiai H, Terakawa N. Low-dose oral contraceptive pill for dysmenorrhea associated with endometriosis: a placebo-controlled, double-blind, randomized trial. Fertil Steril. 2008;90(5):1583-8.

16. Vercellini P, Frontino G, De Giorgi O, Pietropaolo G, Pasin R, Crosignani PG. Continuous use of an oral contraceptive for endometriosis-associated recurrent dysmenorrhea that does not respond to a cyclic pill regimen. Fertil Steril. 2003;80(3):560-3.

17. Brown J, Kives S, Akhtar M. Progestagens and anti-progestagens for pain associated with endometriosis. Cochrane Database Syst Rev. 2012;(3):CD002122.

18. Ferreira RA, Vieira CS, Rosa-E-Silva JC, Rosa-e-Silva AC, Nogueira AA, Ferriani RA. Effects of the levonorgestrel-releasing intrauterine system on cardiovascular risk markers in patients with endometriosis: a comparative study with the GnRH analogue. Contraception. 2010;81(2):117-22.

19. Petta CA, Ferriani RA, Abrao MS, Hassan D, Rosa E Silva JC, Podgaec S, et al. Randomized clinical trial of a levonorgestrel-releasing intrauterine system and a depot GnRH analogue for the treatment of chronic pelvic pain in women with endometriosis. Hum Reprod. 2005;20(7):1993-8.

20. Brown J, Pan A, Hart RJ. Gonadotrophin-releasing hormone analogues for pain associated with endometriosis. Cochrane Database Syst Rev. 2010;(12):CD008475.

21. Al Kadri H, Hassan S, Al-Fozan HM, Hajeer A. Hormone therapy for endometriosis and surgical menopause. Cochrane Database Syst Rev. 2009;(1):CD005997.

22. Moghissi KS, Schlaff WD, Olive DL, Skinner MA, Yin H. Goserelin acetate (Zoladex) with or without hormone replacement therapy for the treatment of endometriosis. Fertil Steril. 1998;69(6):1056-62.

23. Barbieri RL. Hormone treatment of endometriosis: the estrogen threshold hypothesis. Am J Obstet Gynecol. 1992;166(2):740-5.

24. Ferrero S, Gillott DJ, Venturini PL, Remorgida V. Use of aromatase inhibitors to treat endometriosis-related pain symptoms: a systematic review. Reprod Biol Endocrinol. 2011;9:89.

25. Hart RJ, Hickey M, Maouris P, Buckett W. Excisional surgery versus ablative surgery for ovarian endometriomata. Cochrane Database Syst Rev. 2008;(2):CD004992.

26. Busacca M, Riparini J, Somigliana E, Oggioni G, Izzo S, Vignali M, et al. Postsurgical ovarian failure after laparoscopic excision of bilateral endometriomas. Am J Obstet Gynecol. 2006;195(2):421-5.

27. Chapron C, Santulli P, de Ziegler D, Noel JC, Anaf V, Streuli I. Ovarian endometrioma: severe pelvic pain is associated with deeply infiltrating endometriosis. Hum Reprod. 2012;27(3):702-11.

28. Meuleman C, Tomassetti C, D'Hoore A, Van Cleynenbreugel B, Penninckx F, Vergote I, et al. Surgical treatment of deeply infiltrating endometriosis with colorectal involvement. Hum Reprod Update. 2011;17(3):311-26.

29. Vercellini P, Crosignani PG, Somigliana E, Berlanda N, Barbara G, Fedele L. Medical treatment for rectovaginal endometriosis: what is the evidence? Hum Reprod. 2009;24(10):2504-14.

30. Kondo W, Bourdel N, Tamburro S, Cavoli D, Jardon K, Rabischong B, et al. Complications after surgery for deeply infiltrating pelvic endometriosis. BJOG. 2011;118(3):292-8.

31. Jatan AK, Solomon MJ, Young J, Cooper M, Pathma-Nathan N. Laparoscopic management of rectal endometriosis. Dis Colon Rectum. 2006;49(2):169-74.

32. Martin DC. Hysterectomy for treatment of pain associated with endometriosis. J Minim Invasive Gynecol. 2006;13(6):566-72.
33. Namnoum AB, Hickman TN, Goodman SB, Gehlbach DL, Rock JA. Incidence of symptom recurrence after hysterectomy for endometriosis. Fertil Steril. 1995;64(5):898-902.
34. Proctor M, Latthe P, Farquhar C, Khan K, Johnson N. Surgical interruption of pelvic nerve pathways for primary and secondary dysmenorrhoea. Cochrane Database Syst Rev. 2005;(4):CD001896.
35. Barnard ND, Scialli AR, Hurlock D, Bertron P. Diet and sex-hormone binding globulin dysmenorrhea, and premenstrual symptoms. Obstet Gynecol. 2000;95(2):245-50.
36. Cavaggioni G, Lia C, Resta S, Antonielli T, Benedetti Panici P, et al. Are mood and anxiety disorders and alexithymia associated with endometriosis? A preliminary study. Biomed Res Int. 2014;2014:786830.

# CHAPTER 5

# Surgical Management of Endometriosis

*Gaurav S Desai, Shyam V Desai, Priyanka Honavar*

## INTRODUCTION

Endometriosis is a condition that amounts to considerable concern for the woman. Treatment of endometriosis involves a multimodality approach which includes medication and lifestyle modification. In some instances, surgery is used to confirm diagnosis and remove disease pathology, particularly to provide pain relief or improved fertility. Difficulties in establishing a final diagnosis of endometriosis due to the wide variety of clinical practice in the management result in either delayed or suboptimal care.[1]

Successful intervention with the correct modality provides relief from sometime debilitating symptoms and achievement of pregnancy if that is an objective.[2] Apart from diagnosis, role of surgery in a case of endometriosis is vital for the management of endometriosis-associated pain, excision of the endometriosis lesions, interruption of pain pathways, treatment of ovarian or deep infiltrating endometriosis and, sometimes, hysterectomy in cases refractory to other lines of management.

Surgery can be done by an open procedure, by laparoscopy or by robotic intervention. Laparoscopy which is the "gold standard" for diagnosis allows not only diagnosis but also direct surgical treatment (see and treat approach), disease staging and has its own advantage over open surgery. Laparoscopy is usually preferred to open surgery as it provides for better cosmesis, shorter hospital stay, and a lower pain scale score. Robotics is an emerging sector and is taking over laparascopic procedures provided trained personnel are available.

Surgical intervention in endometriosis is indicated in the following situations:

- Women with significant pain
- Those women not responding to medication or in whom medication does not reverse disease burden
- Women who have known contraindications to medication
- Acute adnexal event, e.g., ovarian torsion or rupture
- Invasive pathology involving urinary bladder and ureter, bowel or pelvic nerves
- Ovarian endometrioma

**Flowchart 1:** Surgical intervention in endometriosis.

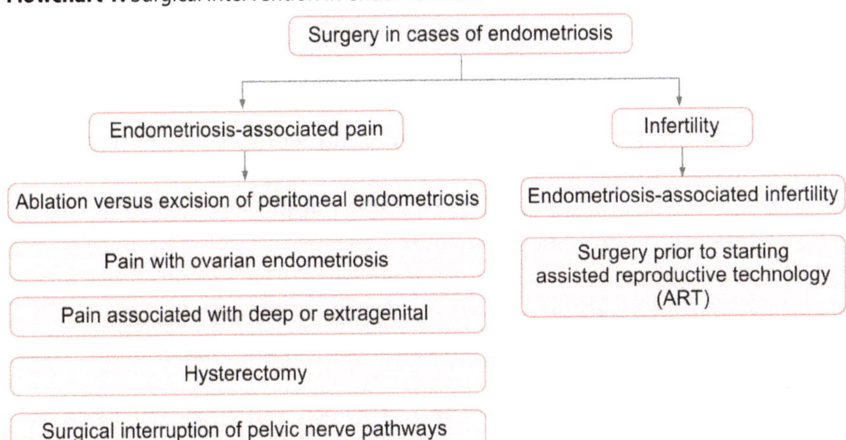


- Women with chronic pelvic pain
- Women seeking fertility.

The intensity of pain associated with the disease does not necessarily correlate with invasiveness rather with the location. Excision, coagulation, LASER vaporization of endometriotic lesions, adhesiolysis or laparoscopic uterosacral nerve ablation (LUNA) are the methods employed depending on the site and extent of the lesions.

Laparotomy and laparoscopy are surgical routes which are effective in removal of endometriosis in the pelvis. Excision of lesions at operative laparoscopy is superior in the treatment of pelvic pain associated with endometriosis in comparison to diagnostic laparoscopy. When endometriosis is identified at laparoscopy, clinicians are recommended to surgically treat endometriosis **(Flowchart 1)**.[3]

## ABLATION VERSUS EXCISION OF ENDOMETRIOSIS

Ablation and excision of peritoneal endometriosis can be considered to reduce endometriosis-associated pain.[4,5] Excision of lesions should be preferred with regard to the possibility of retrieving samples for histology.[6] Excision of endometriosis implants also reduces recurrence rates and pain scores. This is because endometriosis lesions coexist with underlying fibrosis. This underlying fibrosis blunts the response to medication and needs surgical excision. In women seeking fertility, extensive resection requires placement of adhesion barriers.

## PAIN WITH OVARIAN ENDOMETRIOSIS

Cystectomy is superior to laser vaporization[7] and drainage and coagulation in women with ovarian endometrioma, especially if >3 cm with regard to the recurrence of endometriosis-associated pain and the recurrence of endometrioma.[8] The Cochrane Database provides evidence that laparoscopic excision is superior to laparoscopic ablation of ovarian endometriosis for pelvic pain.

Practitioners usually resort to giving oral medication in patients with small endometriomas. In those patients where there is an increase in size or no response to oral medicines, a surgical approach is undertaken. In case of bilateral endometriomas stuck together, i.e., kissing ovaries, the surgeon will separate the ovaries and create a space between the ovaries, the rectum posteriorly and the ureter on each side. Prevention of adhesions is recommended and in some case, use of a T-lift device for the ovaries is done.

## PAIN ASSOCIATED WITH DEEP INFILTRATING ENDOMETRIOSIS

Can extend below the peritoneum and involves the uterosacral ligaments, ureters, the rectum as well as the bladder and the lateral pelvic wall structures. Presence of nodules and fibrosis entails surgical removal. Colorectal involvement can occur and the management involves superficial shaving or resection of the deep endometriosis nodules. It reduces endometriosis-associated pain and improves quality-of-life.[9,10] These surgeries should be performed at centers that offer multidisciplinary services like urosurgery, gastrointestinal surgery, colorectal surgery and imaging. A good preoperative plan includes accurate diagnosis with imaging modalities such as ultrasono-graphy and MRI. Further, a good bowel preparation the night prior is needed for rectovaginal endometriosis. Determining location and depth of infiltration of nodules is of paramount importance. Additionally, having a surgeon on standby helps in surgery.

The goal is to remove the disease and at the same time reduce the morbidity associated with extensive surgery. Surgical techniques which are less extensive are shaving which aims to preserve the intestinal wall and discoid resection instead of segmental resection which maintains bowel continuity. Brouwer and Woods concluded that incomplete dissection of the rectal wall had a five times increased risk of recurrence as compared to full thickness excision and a 10-fold increase in comparison to segmental resection.

A French study with over 1,000 participants found conservative surgery, i.e., shaving had a better quality-of-life than surgery involving excision of the entire rectal wall. Rate of complications such as rectal fistulas is more common with more invasive bowel resection. Additionally, late complications from bowel resection can result from rectal denervation and bowel stenosis. Voiding and defecation should be assessed both preoperatively and postoperatively based on subjective scoring systems.

A laparoscopic approach in difficult cases of extensive disease involves dissection from normal appearing area, following the vessels when finding a plane is not easy, using mesentery of bowel as a guide for plane, releasing the peritoneum and mobilizing the ureters till the tunnel which helps in opening up the deep pararectal space when uterosacrals are fibrosed. The lateral and posterior rectal plane, deep pararectal plane and paravesical plane are usually free in endometriosis and can be used to facilitate surgical objectives.

## PAIN IN EXTRAGENITAL ENDOMETRIOSIS

Symptoms of endometriosis depend on the site of the disease. Cyclical symptoms may be the only clue that leads to the suspicion of endometriosis. Diagnosis is made by histopathological confirmation which is essential to exclude other pathology and malignancy. Site-specific imaging and endoscopic investigations specific to the location may also be used. Consider surgical removal of symptomatic extragenital endometriosis, when possible, to relieve symptoms.[11-15] Appendicular endometriosis is treated by appendectomy.

Surgical management of bladder endometriosis involves excision of the disease and closure of bladder wall defect. Ureteral lesions can be excised after stenting the ureter, segmental excision with end-to-end anastomosis or reimplantation can be done if intrinsic lesions or obstruction is noted. Endometriosis of the abdominal wall and perineum is treated by complete excision.[11-15]

Rarely, the sciatic and other pelvic nerves may cause excruciating pain and can be managed with surgical excision of the disease. In case of thoracic endometriosis, insertion of a chest tube drain helps in case of pneumothorax or hemothorax, followed by chemical pleurodesis or pleurectomy, if recurrence is noted. Persistent hemoptysis due to parenchymal lesions may be treated by lobectomy, segmentectomy or bronchoscopic laser ablation.[16] Damage to nerves during surgery to treat deep infiltrating endometriosis can lead to functional impairments including voiding difficulty. Knowledge of pelvic neuroanatomy and a risk–benefit analysis of the procedure to be undertaken is, therefore, necessary, and management should be individualized.

## HYSTERECTOMY FOR ENDOMETRIOSIS-ASSOCIATED PAIN

Hysterectomy with removal of the ovaries and visible endometriosis lesions can be offered to women who have finished childbearing and in those where conservative medical treatment has little or no effect. Women should be informed that hysterectomy will not necessarily cure the symptoms or the disease, especially for areas of microscopic implants, which could be missed out during the surgery. Hysterectomy may benefit patients with pelvic pain as a result of endometriosis even with ovarian preservation. Shakiba et al.

observed that by 2 years after initial surgery, no further surgery had been required for 80% of the women who had local excision of endometriotic lesions versus 96% of those who underwent hysterectomy with ovaries preserved.

## SURGICAL INTERRUPTION OF PELVIC NERVE PATHWAYS

Another option as a part of surgical management is interruption of nerve pathways, i.e., alteration of pain perception with either LUNA or presacral neurectomy (PSN). LUNA should not be done in addition to conservative surgery to reduce endometriosis-associated pain, since it does not offer any additional benefit over surgery alone.[17] PSN requires a high degree of skill and is a potentially hazardous though effective additional procedure to conservative surgery in reducing endometriosis-associated midline pain.[18] It is associated with increased risk of bleeding, constipation, urinary urgency and painless first stage of labor and for these reasons, not advocated.

## PREOPERATIVE HORMONAL MEDICATION FOR ENDOMETRIOSIS-ASSOCIATED PAIN

Preoperative medical treatment with gonadotrophin-releasing hormone (GnRH) analogs can facilitate surgery by reducing inflammation and vascularization of endometriosis lesions and adhesions. Medical treatment should be offered before surgery to women with painful symptoms with the intention of reducing pain before, not after surgery.[19] Recurrence of 30% is seen for ovarian endometriomas after laparoscopic excision. Patients may benefit from postoperative hormonal suppression.

## ROLE OF SURGERY IN SECONDARY PREVENTION OF RECURRENCE FOR TREATED ENDOMETRIOSIS

Surgeons should perform ovarian cystectomy instead of drainage and electrocoagulation for the secondary prevention of associated dysmenorrhea, dyspareunia and nonmenstrual pelvic pain.[8]

In infertile women with mild-to-moderate endometriosis, operative laparoscopy either excision or ablation including adhesiolysis rather than diagnostic laparoscopy only should be performed to increase the pregnancy rates.[20,21] The goal of operative laparoscopy lies in the restoration of tubo-ovarian anatomy in this subset of patients.

Carbon dioxide ($CO_2$) laser vaporization of endometriosis is preferred over monopolar electrocoagulation as it results in a higher cumulative spontaneous pregnancy rate.[22] In cases of ovarian endometrioma, excision of the capsule instead of drainage and electrocoagulation of the wall is recommended.[8] Women with an endometrioma should be explained the risks of reduced ovarian function after surgery and the possible loss of part or whole of the ovary. The anti-Müllerian hormone (AMH) and antral follicle count (AFC) done preoperatively serve as a reference.

In the situation where there is a difficulty in attaining the plane of cleavage, a shortcut on the ovarian tissue may reveal the space between the cyst and the capsule. Surgeons frequently resort to electrosurgery to achieve hemostasis after cystectomy. This may reduce antral follicles leading to a poor ovarian reserve. Alternatives to reducing blood loss include use of vasopressin and hemostatic agents.

Decision to proceed with the surgery should be considered carefully if the woman has had previous ovarian surgery. In stage III and IV endometriosis, clinicians can consider operative laparoscopy instead of expectant management to increase spontaneous pregnancy rates.[23,24] Operative laparoscopy with adhesiolysis and freeing of adherent ovaries allows in vitro fertilization (IVF) specialists easy access during egg retrieval.

## SURGERY PRIOR TO STARTING ASSISTED REPRODUCTIVE TECHNOLOGY WITH PERITONEAL, OVARIAN AND DEEP ENDOMETRIOSIS

In infertile women with AFS/ASRM (American Fertility Society/American Society for Reproductive Medicine) stage I or II endometriosis, complete surgical removal of peritoneal endometriosis at laparoscopy may improve live birth rate prior to assisted reproduction.[25] Surgical therapy is needed for peritoneal endometriosis, ovarian endometrioma (ablation, cystectomy, aspiration) and for deep endometriosis prior to assisted reproductive technology (ART). In women keen on conception with small endometriomas, i.e., less than 3 cm, evidence does not support cystectomy prior to ART for improved pregnancy rates. In women with endometriomas more than 3 cm in size, a cystectomy prior to ART can help to improve associated pain or the access to follicles.

Women presenting with endometrioma should be counselled regarding the risks of reduced ovarian function following surgery and the possible loss of the ovary. The decision to proceed with surgery should be considered carefully if the woman has had previous ovarian surgery.[8,26,27] The effectiveness of surgical excision of deep nodular lesions before treatment with assisted reproductive technologies in women with endometriosis-associated infertility is not well-established with regard to reproductive outcome.

## ROLE OF SURGERY IN ASYMPTOMATIC ENDOMETRIOSIS

Most lesions are seen incidentally on laparoscopy without the woman having any symptoms. Surgical excision or ablation (and its risks of damage to the bowel, bladder, ureter and blood vessels) for incidental asymptomatic endometriosis cannot be encouraged, because of doubtful benefits. Furthermore, the risk that asymptomatic minimal disease will become symptomatic is low.[28] Nonetheless excision of an implant can ascertain histopathological diagnosis.

## CONCLUSION

Endometriosis can have a varied presentation with both genital and extragenital symptoms. Each case needs a thorough evaluation, staging, apt diagnosis and the best management possible.

When one resorts to surgical management for any indication, patient selection, surgical method and route selection, counseling and follow-up will always form an integral part of patient care.

## REFERENCES


1. Kennedy S, Bergqvist A, Chapron C, D'Hooghe T, Dunselman G, Greb R, et al. ESHRE guideline for the diagnosis and treatment of endometriosis. Hum Reprod. 2005;20(10):2698-704.
2. Leyland N, Casper R, Laberge P, Singh SS, SOGC. Endometriosis: diagnosis and management. J Obstet Gynaecol Can. 2010;32(7 Suppl 2):S1-32.
3. Jacobson TZ, Duffy JM, Barlow D, Koninckx PR, Garry R. Laparoscopic surgery for pelvic pain associated with endometriosis. Cochrane Database Syst Rev. 2009; (4):CD001300.
4. Healey M, Ang WC, Cheng C. Surgical treatment of endometriosis: a prospective randomized double-blinded trial comparing excision and ablation. Fertil Steril. 2010;94(7):2536-40.
5. Wright J, Lotfallah H, Jones K, Lovell D. A randomized trial of excision versus ablation for mild endometriosis. Fertil Steril. 2005;83(6):1830-6.
6. NICE (2017). Endometriosis: diagnosis and management. NICE guideline [NG73]. [online] Available from: https://www.nice.org.uk/guidance/ng73. [Last accessed October, 2020].
7. Carmona F, Martínez-Zamora MA, Rabanal A, Martínez-Román S, Balasch J. Ovarian cystectomy versus laser vaporization in the treatment of ovarian endometriomas: a randomized clinical trial with a five-year follow-up. Fertil Steril. 2011;96(1):251-4.
8. Hart RJ, Hickey M, Maouris P, Buckett W. Excisional surgery versus ablative surgery for ovarian endometriomata. Cochrane Database Syst Rev. 2008;(2):CD004992.
9. De Cicco C, Corona R, Schonman R, Mailova K, Ussia A, Koninckx P. Bowel resection for deep endometriosis: a systematic review. BJOG. 2011;118(3):285-91.
10. Meuleman C, Tomassetti C, D'Hoore A, Van Cleynenbreugel B, Penninckx F, Vergote I, et al. Surgical treatment of deeply infiltrating endometriosis with colorectal involvement. Hum Reprod Update. 2011;17(3):311-26.
11. Liang CC, Tsai CC, Chen TC, Soong YK. Management of perineal endometriosis. Int J Gynaecol Obstet. 1996;53(3):261-5.
12. Marinis A, Vassiliou J, Kannas D, Theodosopoulos TK, Kondi-Pafiti A, Kairi E, et al. Endometriosis mimicking soft tissue tumors: diagnosis and treatment. Eur J Gynaecol Oncol. 2006;27(2):168-70.
13. Nezhat C, Hajhosseini B, King LP. Robotic-assisted laparoscopic treatment of bowel, bladder, and ureteral endometriosis. JSLS. 2011;15(3):387-92.
14. Nissotakis C, Zouros E, Revelos K, Sakorafas GH. Abdominal wall endometrioma: a case report and review of the literature. AORN J. 2010;91(6):730-42.

15. Song JY, Borncamp E, Mehaffey P, Rotman C. Large abdominal wall endometrioma following laparoscopic hysterectomy. JSLS. 2011;15(2):261-3.

16. Nisolle M, Pasleau F, Foidart JM. Extragenital endometriosis. J Gynecol Obstet Biol Reprod (Paris). 2007;36(2):173-8.

17. Endometriosis: diagnosis and management. SOGC clinical practice guideline. SOGC. 2010;244:S2.

18. Proctor ML, Latthe PM, Farquhar CM, Khan KS, Johnson NP. Surgical interruption of pelvic nerve pathways for primary and secondary dysmenorrhoea. Cochrane Database Syst Rev. 2005;(4):CD001896.

19. Furness S, Yap C, Farquhar C, Cheong YC. Pre and post-operative medical therapy for endometriosis surgery. Cochrane Database Syst Rev. 2004:CD003678.

20. Jacobson TZ, Duffy JM, Barlow D, Farquhar C, Koninckx PR, Olive D. Laparoscopic surgery for subfertility associated with endometriosis. Cochrane Database Syst Rev. 2010;20(1):CD001398.

21. Nowroozi K, Chase JS, Check JH, Wu CH. The importance of laparoscopic coagulation of mild endometriosis in infertile women. Int J Fertil. 1987;32(6):442-4.

22. Chang FH, Chou HH, Soong YK, Chang MY, Lee CL, Lai YM. Efficacy of isotopic $13CO_2$ laser laparoscopic evaporation in the treatment of infertile patients with minimal and mild endometriosis: a life table cumulative pregnancy rates study. J Am Assoc Gynecol Laparosc. 1997;4(2):219-23.

23. Nezhat C, Crowgey S, Nezhat F. Videolaseroscopy for the treatment of endometriosis associated with infertility. Fertil Steril. 1989;51(2):237-40.

24. Vercellini P, Fedele L, Aimi G, De Giorgi O, Consonni D, Crosignani PG. Reproductive performance, pain recurrence and disease relapse after conservative surgical treatment for endometriosis: the predictive value of the current classification system. Hum Reprod. 2006;21(10):2679-85.

25. Opøien HK, Fedorcsak P, Byholm T, Tanbo T. Complete surgical removal of minimal and mild endometriosis improves outcome of subsequent IVF/ICSI treatment. Reprod Biomed Online. 2011;23(3):389-95.

26. Benschop L, Farquhar C, van der Poel N, Heineman MJ. Interventions for women with endometrioma prior to assisted reproductive technology. Cochrane Database Syst Rev. 2010;(11):CD008571.

27. Donnez J, Wyns C, Nisolle M. Does ovarian surgery for endometriomas impair the ovarian response to gonadotropin? Fertil Steril. 2001;76(4):662-5.

28. Moen MH, Stokstad T. A long-term follow-up study of women with asymptomatic endometriosis diagnosed incidentally at sterilization. Fertil Steril. 2002;78(4):773-6.

# CHAPTER 6

# Newer Molecules in Endometriosis

*Anuradha Khanna, Shikha Sachan, Dhivya Sethuraman*

## INTRODUCTION

Endometriosis, histologically defined as the presence of endometrium-like tissue—glands and stroma—that develops outside of the uterine cavity, is still an enigmatic disease responsible for pelvic pain and infertility in reproductive age group. Studies suggest a prevalence of 0.5–5% in fertile and 25–40% in infertile women.[1]

## OVERVIEW OF PATHOGENESIS

The Sampson theory of retrograde menstruation and ectopic implantation of endometrium is one of the most plausible pathology of endometriosis. Retrograde menstruation is a common phenomenon as demonstrated during laparoscopy,[2-5] but endometriosis is also believed to develop de novo or by metaplasia of celomic pluripotent mesothelial cells lining the peritoneum.[2,5-7] Another theory which proposes activation of embryonic rests of endometrial tissues as etiology for endometriosis goes by the name of mullerianosis. However, none of this theory explains presence of endometriosis outside the peritoneal cavity; for this, it was proposed that endometrium cells can travel as microemboli and metastases to different locations by hematogenous or lymphatic route. None of the theories fully explain the occurrence of endometriosis and hence is not exclusive. Grossly during operative interventions, we see three phenotypes which can be found exclusively or together—(1) Peritoneal implants which may be red vesicle like, powder burn areas or clear vesicle like, (2) Deeply infiltrating endometriosis, most commonly seen in rectovaginal fossa in which endometriotic pathology extends more than 5 mm beneath the peritoneum, and (3) Ovarian endometrioma.

It perplexed the scientist that the phenomena responsible for etiopathogenesis of endometriosis are found in most of the women but why is that only few develop endometriosis. While the genetic basis of endometriosis is still a potential research area, it is believed that various inherent host factors at molecular level are involved in the development of lesions. These include dysregulation of estrogen hormone and receptors, predominance of beta subtypes of estrogen receptor (ERβ) over alpha (ERα) subtypes[8,9] and relative progesterone resistance due to less formation of progesterone receptors (PR).[10-12] This helps in proliferation of endometriotic tissue outside uterus as well. Women with endometriosis are known to have impaired immune system response; in addition to that, ectopic endometrial tissues have decreased expression of metalloproteinases, CD36 and increased production of dissolved intercellular adhesion molecule 1,[12] which help them in avoiding destruction by apoptotic and phagocytosis mechanisms. Angiogenic activity is seen increased due to overproduction of interleukin (IL)-1, IL-6, IL-8, monocyte chemoattractant protein 1, RANTES, tumor necrosis factor (TNF)-$\alpha$ and TNF-$\beta$, and the inflammation caused by them.[12,13]

Since the eutopic and ectopic endometrium have different receptor expression, angiogenic activity and different inflammatory milieu, it creates difficulties in the development of new drug therapies and treatments.

## MEDICAL MANAGEMENT OF ENDOMETRIOSIS

Medical therapy often represents the first-line management for women with endometriosis, aiming to ameliorate pain symptoms and to prevent postsurgical disease recurrence. It is usually used for suppression of endometriosis and associated inflammatory process. The choice of the therapy is based on several factors, such as age of the patients, intensity and characteristics of pain, preference of the patients, desire to conceive, and presence of comorbidities, costs, route of administration and impact of the endometriosis on work capacity, sexual function and quality-of-life. Therapies which have minimal side effects, which can be used for a longer duration, and are less costly are used.

Till now, medical therapies have focused on suppression of inflammatory reaction, suppressing endometrium by increasing serum progesterone level or decreasing estrogen level. Most commonly used drugs are combined oral contraceptive (COC), and gonadotrophin-releasing hormone (GnRH) agonist. The aim of these conventional therapies is suppression of endometriotic implants.[14] Traditionally, COCs and nonsteroidal anti-inflammatory drugs (NSAIDs) have been the first-line treatment for patients with endometriosis, but currently, progestins are increasingly and successfully employed as monotherapy, being efficacious and well-tolerated for long period of time. These hormonal compounds are efficacious in controlling symptoms in about two-third of women. Second-line therapy is represented by GnRH agonists, which have a less favorable tolerability profile[15] **(Table 1)**.

Medical therapies, aiming at suppression of endometriotic implants by creating hypoestrogenic environment, cause significant side effects. There are also chances of high relapse rate after discontinuation of an optimal therapy; also, many of these therapies are too costly. Hence, the need of newer

**Table 1:** Agents for the pharmacologic management of endometriosis-associated pain.

| Agent | Dose | Route | Dosing frequency | Common side effects |
|---|---|---|---|---|
| Combined oral contraceptives | 30–35 µg ethinylestradiol, plus progestin | Oral | Daily (cyclic or continuous) | Irregular bleeding, weight gain, bloating, breast tension and headache |
| **Androgens** | | | | |
| Danazol | 400–800 mg | Oral | Daily (duration limited to 6 months by side effects) | Androgenic/ anabolic (weight gain, fluid retention, breast atrophy, acne, oily skin, hot flashes and hirsutism) |
| Gonadotropin-releasing hormone (GnRH) agonists | | | Duration limited to 6 months due to BMD effects | |
| Leuprolide | 1 mg/day | SC injection | Daily | Hypoestrogenic (hot flashes, vaginal dryness, emotional lability, loss of libido and BMD decline) |
| Leuprolide depot | 3.75 mg | IM injection | Monthly | |
| | 11.75 mg | IM injection | Every 3 months | |
| Triptorelin | 3 mg | IM injection | Monthly | |
| Triptorelin depot | 11.25 mg | IM injection | Every 3 months | |
| Goserelin | 3.6 mg | SC implant | Monthly | |
| Buserelin | 300–400 µg | Intranasal | Tid | |
| Nafarelin | 200–400 µg | Intranasal | Bid | |
| **Progestins** | | | | |
| Dydrogesterone | 60 mg | Oral | 12 days per cycle* | |
| Gestrinone | 2.5–5 mg | Oral | Daily/twice weekly | |

*Contd...*

*Contd...*

| Agent | Dose | Route | Dosing frequency | Common side effects |
|---|---|---|---|---|
| Megestrol acetate | 40 mg | Oral | Daily | Irregular bleeding, weight gain, bloating and edema |
| Norethindrone acetate | 5 mg[†] | Oral | Daily | |
| MPA | 30 mg | Oral | Daily | |
| DMPA-IM 150[‡] | 150 mg | IM injection | Every 3 months | |
| DMPA-SC 104[‡] | 104 mg | SC injection | Every 3 months | |

(BMD: bone mineral density; DMPA: depot medroxyprogesterone acetate;
IM: intramuscular; MPA: medroxyprogesterone acetate; SC: subcutaneous)
*During the luteal phase.
[†]Starting dose, with gradual dose escalation.
[‡]Also with transient BMD decline.

drugs aiming at the etiopathogenesis and specific molecular mechanisms to overcome these factors.[8,13,15,16]

Apart from these traditional treatment methods, there are several newer molecules which are now under research to tailor-made the medical management of endometriosis. These are listed later.

## DIENOGEST

Traditionally, progesterone derivatives have been used for treating endometriosis. Progestins (synthetic progestogens) inhibit endometrial tissue growth by causing initial decidualization and then atrophy. Additional proposed mechanisms of action include suppression of matrix metalloproteinases, a class of enzymes important in the growth and implantation of ectopic endometrium, and inhibition of angiogenesis. Dienogest is 19-nortestosterone derivative with strong progestin effect on endometrium, a short plasma half-life of approximately 9 hours, and higher bioavailability. It does not interfere with p450 cytochrome in the liver, has moderate effect on gonadotropin secretion inhibition, and also antiandrogenic activity. Dienogest 2 mg/day has been shown to decrease the concentration of inflammatory proteins associated with aromatase activity, prostaglandin E2 (PGE2) and cyclo-oxygenase (COX)-2 by significantly inhibiting the expression of genes. It has also shown to decrease resistance to progesterone by altering progesterone and estrogen receptor ratio, as it increases the progesterone receptor $\beta/\alpha$ ratio, and decreases the estrogen receptor $\beta/\alpha$ ratio.[12,17,18] Dienogest is increasingly being recognized as single-drug therapy for endometriosis in several countries.[12,19,20] On prolonged administration, it has lower decrease in estrogen level or negative impact on bone mass when compared with GnRH agonists; however, the relief of symptoms provided is similar. The most frequent side effects are breast pain (4.2%), nausea (3.0%), and irritability (2.4%).[12]

## Aromatase Inhibitor

The enzyme aromatase P450 plays an important role in the conversion of androstenedione and testosterone to estrone (E1) and estradiol (E2) in endometrium, and was found to be expressed more in patient with endometriosis, while it was negligible in healthy women. With this etiopathogenesis in mind, many researchers have investigated the role of third-generation nonsteroidal (type 2) aromatase inhibitors (AIs) such as letrozole and anastrozole.

Aromatase inhibitors are used in severe, refractory endometriosis-related pain in conjunction with progestogen, COC, or GnRH agonist. AIs directly decrease aromatase activity in endometriotic tissue and decrease estrogen level, which leads to suppression of COX-2 activity and decreased PGE2 level, this halts the self-propagation of endometriotic implants.[12,21,22] When given to premenopausal women dosage of 0.5 mg decreases estrogen up to 97–99%.[12] The third-generation triazole derivatives of AIs like anastrazole, letrozole and exemestane have recommended daily dose of 1 mg, 2.5 mg and 25 mg, respectively. Their effects are usually reversible, potent and selective, making it a good choice over earlier generations.[12,23] AIs, significantly, are superior in preventing postoperative recurrence when compared to GnRH or danazol, within 6 months' period. Currently, the European Society of Human Reproduction and Embryology (ESHRE) guidelines only suggest the administration of AIs in combination with COCs, progestins or GnRH-agonists in women with rectovaginal endometriosis, refractory to other medical or surgical treatment. Newer trials are testing anastrozole as vaginal ring and suppository for rectovaginal endometriosis.[24] Side effects are mild headache, joint pain or stiffness, nausea, diarrhea, hot flashes, mild bone density decrease, but long-term use can lead to formation of functional ovarian cyst.

## Gonadotrophin-releasing Hormone Antagonist

Gonadotrophin-releasing hormone antagonists cause a competitive blockage of the GnRH receptor. Thus, they immediately suppress the production of luteinizing hormone (LH) and follicle-stimulating hormone (FSH) and, consequently, they inhibit the secretion of gonadal steroid hormones without inducing a flare-up effect (different from GnRH-agonists). The reduction in the amount of circulating estrogens without their complete suppression improves endometriosis related pain symptoms causing lower estrogen-related adverse effects. GnRH-antagonists can be administered by subcutaneous injections (Cetrorelix) or by oral administration [Elagolix, (ELX)]. Symptom relief and adverse events such as vasomotor phenomena, vaginal atrophy, and bone loss are also dose-dependent. GnRH antagonists provide a treatment option for women who do not respond to NSAIDs, estrogen–progestin contraceptives, or progestins.

In trials, it was found that GnRH antagonist elagolix (150 mg once daily or 200 mg twice daily) significantly reduced endometriosis-related dysmenorrhea and noncyclic pelvic pain, which was comparable to DMPA injection. The most common side effects are hot flush, nausea, headache, and amenorrhea. Elagolix causes a mild decrease in axial bone density, baseline in bone mineral density (BMD) at the lumbar spine, femoral neck, and total hip, which was significantly lower after 6 months of treatment. The rate of pregnancy increases by 5% at a dose of 150 mg/day. No teratogenic effect was found from elagolix treatment.[12,24] The FDA has approved elagolix (*Orilissa*), the first drug developed for the treatment of moderate-to-severe pain from endometriosis in July 2018. It is first oral GnRH agonist in American market.

Relugolix is another orally available nonpeptide GnRH antagonist, under investigation for the treatment of endometriosis. While add-back therapy is recommended with the use of GnRH agonists, up to now, no study assessed the use of add-back therapy in patients receiving GnRH antagonists.

## Selective Estrogen Receptor Modulator

The selective estrogen receptor modulators (SERMs) are agents that have different agonistic and antagonistic action on endometrial receptor located in different organs. SERMs avoid the side effect of estrogen by having agonistic effects on bones, central nervous system and blood vessels while having antagonistic action on endometrium. Example of selective estrogen receptor modulator are tamoxifen, raloxifene, and bazedoxifene (BZA). In studies conducted on animals, raloxifene reduced the size of lesions similar to the effect of AI anastrozole. In humans, the results are still inconclusive and require further research.

Preclinical studies showed that administration of BZA (3 mg/kg/day) or BZA-conjugated estrogen combination causes regression of endometriotic lesions, decreased estrogen receptor expression, and reduced expression of various genes involved in tissue proliferation. SR-16234 is another experimental SERM with antagonistic activity on ER$\alpha$ and partial agonistic activity on ER$\beta$. Differently from other SERMs (such raloxifene and bazedoxifene), SR-16234 seems to have a purer antagonist activity against

ERα; this characteristic may justify its hypothetic effectiveness for treating endometriosis.

## Selective Progesterone Receptor Modulator

As with SERM, selective progesterone receptor modulators (SPRMs) bind to progesterone receptors in various tissues causing both agonistic and antagonistic action, so selective progesterone receptor modulator (SPRMs). So, the ideal SPRM for therapy would be the one which has antagonist action on endometrium bringing down its thickness, with loss of mitotic activity and increased stromal density, but retains the protective effects of estrogen on bone and cardiovascular systems. Various animal studies have revealed that suppression effect on hypothalamus–pituitary–gonadal axis is seen more with SPRM rather than inhibiting ovarian estrogen production suppression. SPRM being investigated for treatment of endometriosis are asoprisnil, asoprisnil ecamate and ulipristal. In animal studies, asoprisnil and asoprisnil ecamate have successfully suppressed endometrial proliferation resulting in amenorrhea and endometrial atrophy, while ulipristal has shown promise by reducing endometriotic focci by at least 50% and a decrease in the number of cells exhibiting proliferative activity.

In humans, administration of ulipristal acetate (doses 10, 50 or 100 mg) has shown to decrease endometrial thickness and consequently cause endometrial atrophy. Histopathologically, on treatment, the glandular architecture shows mixed secretory and proliferative characteristics.

## Antitumor Necrosis Factor-α

Tumor necrosis factor-α is a proinflammatory molecule, which plays an important role in etiopathogenesis of endometriosis. It potentiates other inflammatory molecules and helps in autopropagation of endometriotic endometrium, and so anti-TNF-α monoclonal antibodies (infliximab) or soluble TNF-α receptors (etanercept, TNF recombinant human protein bindings) are a plausible treatment approach for endometriosis. Anti-TNF-α molecules, however, do not have a very important role in infertility associated with endometriosis; although studies have shown it inhibits the development of lesions and sometimes causes the regression of existing lesion. Side effects may include milder one like headache and allergic reactions during intravenous administration, or more sinister which are associated with long-term therapy with serious infections and tuberculosis reactivation.

## Enzyme Inhibitors

Steroid sulfatase (STS) enzyme has an important role in formation of biologically active estrogen from inactive steroid sulfate in endometrium. The enzyme catalyze the hydrolysis of estrone sulfate and dehydroepiandrosterone sulfate (DHEAS) to their unconjugated forms, estrone and DHEA, respectively. Many researchers have correlated the severity of disease with activity of STS enzyme and, hence, for this reason, the inhibition of STS enzyme is targeted as therapy of endometriosis.

In addition, unbalanced local activity in ectopic endometrium of the 17β-Hydroxysteroid dehydrogenases (17β-HSDs) converts the low-potent E1 into the high-potent E2 (reducing 17β-HSD1). Estrone 3-O-sulfamate, known as EMATE, has been the first estrogen sulfamate tested. It was chosen for the sulfate group that led to reversible inhibition of ST. The pharmacokinetic profile of the steroid derivative PBRM, a first potent covalent inhibitor of 17β-HSD1 that has no estrogenic activity, has been recently studied in mice with promising results. FOR-6219, a novel HSD 17B1 inhibitor, is being developed for the treatment of endometriosis.

## Biological Therapy

Biological therapy is an emerging therapeutic option based on agents designed to specifically target a biological phenomenon, gene, protein, or group of genes or proteins involved in a specific disease. It mainly includes monoclonal antibodies and tyrosine kinase inhibitors (TKIs) that specifically target critical pathways for cell survival and proliferation as well as specific or nonspecific immune stimulators (antibodies, cytokines, vaccines or cellular therapy). In the last years, gene and DNA repair enzyme inhibitor represent other emerging opportunities in this field. Angiogenesis has a critical role in the development and growth of endometriotic implants; vascular endothelial growth factor (VEGF) is the most important molecule involved in this process and, hence, therapies targeting VEGF are also being developed for the treatment of endometriosis.

## Noninvasive Therapy

### High-intensity Focused Ultrasound

High-intensity focused ultrasound (HIFU) is a new technique that utilizes the principle that when ultrasonic waves are focused on a certain point, high intensity acoustic energy will be absorbed and then converted into heat at the designed focal point, resulting in thermal coagulation. HIFU needs precision and focus, so is performed under the guidance of ultrasound (USgHIFU) or magnetic resonance imaging. HIFU is already being used in treatment of adenomyosis with significant improvement of clinical symptoms. So, it was proposed as a futuristic treatment for ablating the ectopic endometrial implants in endometriosis. However, there are certain challenges in using this technology, i.e., it is a time-consuming procedure in certain cases and, since the precision is mandatory, no movement of patient is allowed making regional anesthesia part of procedure. Also, the ultrasonic waves cannot penetrate hollow viscera. Severe complications ever reported are postprocedure vaginal bleeding, and unexplained tumor enlargement that causes discomfort.

## CONCLUSION

Endometriosis is a gynecologic disorder which causes severe morbidity by interfering with woman's day-to-day life. Medical therapy is only suppressive but offers a suitable choice in women by improving their quality-of-life. Dienogest, AI, and GnRH antagonists are the newer drugs with good tolerance and safety and are emerging as effective treatment of endometriosis. SERM and SPRM are mostly still in phase I and II clinical trials, results of which are still showing inconsistent results. Anti-TNF-$\alpha$ is still studied in the animal model. HIFU is a promising futuristic treatment. However, it is still a long way until the logistics for making this technology applicable appear.

## REFERENCES


1. Child TJ, Tan SL. Endometriosis, aetiology, pathogenesis and treatment. Drugs. 2001;61(12):1735-50.
2. Honda R, Katabuchi H. Pathological aspect and pathogenesis of endometriosis. In: Harada T (Ed). Endometriosis: Pathogenesis and Treatment. Tokyo: Springer; 2014. pp. 9-18.
3. Schweppe KW, Rabe T, Langhardt M, Woziwodzki J, Petraglia F, Kiesel L. Endometriosis: pathogenesis, diagnosis, and therapeutic options for clinical and ambulatory care. J Reproduktionsmed Endokrinol. 2013;10:102-19.
4. Reis FM, Petraglia F, Taylor RN. Endometriosis: hormone regulation and clinical consequences of chemotaxis and apoptosis. Hum Reprod Update. 2013;19:406-18.
5. Macer ML, Taylor HS. Endometriosis and infertility: a review of the pathogenesis and treatment of endometriosis-associated infertility. Obstet Gynecol Clin North Am. 2012;39:535-49.
6. Ahn SH, Monsanto SP, Miller C, Singh SS, Thomas R, Tayade C. Pathophysiology and immune dysfunction in endometriosis. Biomed Res Int. 2015;2015:795976.
7. Aznaurova YB, Zhumataev MB, Roberts TK, Aliper AM, Zhavoronkov AA. Molecular aspects of development and regulation of endometriosis. Reprod Biol Endocrinol. 2014;12:50.
8. Bulun SE, Cheng YH, Pavone ME, Xue Q, Attar E, Trukhacheva E, et al. Estrogen receptor-beta, estrogen receptor-alpha, and progesterone resistance in endometriosis. Semin Reprod Med. 2010;28:36-43.
9. Bulun SE. Endometriosis. N Engl J Med. 2009;360:268-79.
10. Bulun SE, Monsavais D, Pavone ME, Dyson M, Xue Q, Attar E, et al. Role of estrogen receptor-$\beta$ in endometriosis. Semin Reprod Med. 2012;30:39-45.
11. Maia H Jr, Haddad C, Coelho G, Casoy J. Role of inflammation and aromatase expression in the eutopic endometrium and its relationship with the development of endometriosis. Womens Health (Lond). 2012;8:647-58.
12. Suardika A, Astawa Pemayun TG. New insights on the pathogenesis of endometriosis and novel non-surgical therapies. Novel therapies for endometriosis. J Turk Ger Gynecol Assoc. 2018;19(3):158-64.
13. Herington JL, Bruner-Tran KL, Lucas JA, Osteen KG. Immune interactions in endometriosis. Expert Rev Clin Immunol. 2011;7:611-26.

14. Dhesi AS, Morelli SS. Endometriosis: a role for stem cells. Women's Health (Lond). 2015;11:35-49.
15. Falcone T, Flyckt R. Clinical management of endometriosis. Obstet Gynecol. 2018;131:557-71.
16. Ferrero S, Barra F, Leone Roberti Maggiore U. Current and emerging therapeutics for the management of endometriosis. Drugs. 2018;78(10):995-1012.
17. Bizzarri N, Remorgida V, Leone Roberti Maggiore U, Scala C, Tafi E, Ghirardi V, et al. Dienogest in the treatment of endometriosis. Expert Opin Pharmacother. 2014;15:1889-902.
18. Ruan X, Seeger H, Mueck AO. The pharmacology of dienogest. Maturitas. 2012;71:337-44.
19. Mueck AO. Dienogest: an oral progestogen for the treatment of endometriosis. Expert Rev Obstet Gynecol. 2011;6:5-15.
20. Schindler AE. Dienogest in long-term treatment of endometriosis. Int J Womens Health. 2011;3:175-84.
21. Pavone ME, Bulun SE. Aromatase inhibitors for the treatment of endometriosis. Fertil Steril. 2012;98:1370-9.
22. Agarwal SK, Foster WG. Reduction in endometrioma size with three months of aromatase inhibition and progestin add-back. Biomed Res Int. 2015;2015:878517.
23. Buzdar AU. Pharmacology and pharmacokinetics of the newer generation aromatase inhibitors. Clin Cancer Res. 2003;9:468-72.
24. Barra F, Grandi G, Tantari M, Scala C, Facchinetti F, Ferrero S. A comprehensive review of hormonal and biological therapies for endometriosis: latest developments. Expert Opin Biol Ther. 2019;19(4):343-60.

# CHAPTER 7

# Recurrence and How to Deal?

*T Ramani Devi, S Chitra, N Gayathri*

## INTRODUCTION

Endometriosis is a relatively common disease which affects 11% of women of reproductive age group. It is characterized by extrauterine implantation of endometrial-like tissues triggering chronic inflammatory reaction which clinically manifests with pelvic pain, pelvic mass and infertility. Because the endometrial cells are hormonally influenced, symptoms of endometriosis often worsen during menstrual period. Basically, recurrent endometriosis is a frequently encountered benign disorder, where approximately 30% of patients undergo repeated surgeries. Recurrence occurs either in the form of pelvic pain, which presents as dysmenorrhea, dyspareunia, dyschezia and diffuse abdominal pain. Recurrence of lesion is usually identified in the form of pelvic mass or nodularity detected through clinical examination or imaging techniques. Pain recurrence is more common than lesion recurrence. The rate of recurrence of endometriosis is 20% after 2 years and 40–50% after 5 years in a study by Sun Wei et al. According to the staging of endometriosis, at the end of 2 years, recurrence rate is around 5–7% for stage I and II and 14.3% for stage III and IV. Various studies have suggested recurrence rate between 6 and 67%.[1,2]

## FACTORS AFFECTING RECURRENCE

The risk of recurrence depends on the primary location of lesion. Busacca et al.[3] studied 144 recurrence cases and reported the 4-year recurrence rates as 24.6% for ovarian, 17.8% for peritoneal, 30.6% for deep and 23.7% for peritoneal endometriosis. Eight years' recurrence rates were 42, 24.1, 43.4 and 30.9% respectively.[4]

Li et al. followed up 285 patients for a period of 36 months and reported the following parameters as risk factor for recurrence—bilateral, pelvic involvement of endometriotic lesion, tender nodularity at cul-de-sac, previous surgeries, preoperative [revised American Fertility Society (rAFS)] score and young age.

Body mass index (BMI), age at menarche, parity, previous treatment, age at surgery, intraoperative size of the cyst, and coexistence of myoma are few factors which did not affect the recurrence risk. Severity of the disease and extensiveness of surgery might affect the overall recurrence risk.

Parazzini et al.[5] showed that the advanced stage disease initially had a higher recurrence rate and Busacca et al.[3] reported that young age, deep endometriosis, stage III or IV and interval following surgery were additional risk factors for recurrence **(Table 1)**.

Many authors reported that pregnancy after surgery serves as a protective factor for recurrence as increased progesterone levels suppress the activation and growth of lesions, thereby inhibiting inflammation.[6]

Recurrence mainly develops due to either of the two factors:

1. Newer lesions developing after surgery.
2. Reactivation and persistence of existing lesions. In a study conducted by Vignali et al.,[7] the pain recurrence was 20.5% at the end of 3 years and 43.5% at the end of 5 years, whereas the clinical recurrence rates were 9% and 28%, respectively.

**Table 1:** Risk factors for recurrence of endometriosis.

| Study (year) | Risk factors |
| --- | --- |
| Fedele (2004)<br>Vignali (2005)<br>Vercellini (2006)<br>Liu (2007)<br>Molni A (2014) | Younger age |
| Ghezzi (2001)<br>Jones and Sutton (2002) | Laterality of lesions |
| Waller and Shaw (1993)<br>Busacca (1999)<br>Parazzini (2005)<br>Abbott (2003)<br>Li (2005)<br>Kikuchi (2006)<br>Liu (2007)<br>Moini A (2014) | rAFS stage<br>rAFS > 70<br>rAFS score |
| Saleh and Tulandi (1999)<br>Koga (2006)<br>Moini A (2014) | Size of cyst |
| Renner (2010) | High preoperative pain |
| Bulletti (2001)<br>Fedele (2004)<br>Li (2005) | Absence of pregnancy |
| Koga (2006)<br>Liu (2007) | Previous medical treatment |
| Vignali (2005)<br>Fedele (2000) | Completeness of the first surgery<br>Extend of surgical excision |
| Li (2005) | Painful nodule |
| (rAFS: revised American Fertility Society) | |

## PATHOPHYSIOLOGY

Persistence of retrograde menstruation, high premenstrual uterine tone, frequency, amplitude and incidence of retrograde uterine contractions are few theories behind the development of newer lesions. Lymphovascular involvement could also be another cause for recurrence, most commonly seen in rectovaginal endometriosis.[8] This phenomenon mimics malignancy and may be a reason for recurrence. Apart from this, estrogen receptor (ER) polymorphism, *ERα* P-vull may be responsible for increased propensity of recurrence.

## IMMUNOLOGICAL ROLE FOR RECURRENCE

Natural killer (NK) cell suppression in endometriosis provides a wider environment for recurrence.[9] This depends on few genetic and immunological factors. Treatment (either medically or surgically) reduces only the burden of the disease but does not address the etiological factors. Recurrence due to reactivation is because of increased aromatase expression in the endometriotic lesions, fat, bone, adrenal tissue and in endometrium of endometriotic patients. The cause for this overactivity is that, in endometriosis, the estrogen biosynthesis in peripheral tissue and endometriotic implants by aromatase are not inhibited.

## RISK FACTORS ASSOCIATED WITH RECURRENCE

Although various factors are associated with recurrence, it is still unclear regarding which factor is more predictive. Young age, laterality of lesions and rAFS scores were considered in grouping patients into low-risk group and high-risk group[10] **(Table 2)**.

## RECURRENCE RATE

Recurrence rate is influenced by factors which presents as pain, infertility (symptomatically) or in the form of clinical recurrence (as seen in MRI, USG,

**Table 2:** Low risk and high risk factors associated with recurrence.

| Low risk | High risk |
|---|---|
| rAFS score < 70 | rAFS score > 70 |
| Pregnancy, OCP | Bilateral mass |
| Endometrial ablation | Suboptimal surgery |
| Unilateral lesions | No postoperative medical management |
| Complete surgery | Young age |
| Postoperative medication | Ovarian conservation |
| (OCP: oral contraceptive pill; rAFS: revised American Fertility Society) | |

etc.). Apart from this, recurrence also depends upon the type and extent of pre-existing disease, time of patient's follow-up, surgical expertise and intervention.

## Incidence of Recurrent Endometriosis

Of total, 45% of patients showed pain recurrence 1 year after surgery and 9–15% shows reappearance of disease (by confirmed clinically or by USG). After conservative surgery followed by 6 months medical treatment, 26% had pain which recurred 1 year later and 8% had detectable disease after 1 year.

Clinical recurrence usually presents in the form of endometriotic cysts more than 10 mm in the ovaries. Here, 24% were asymptomatic whereas 76% had flared up symptom recurrence.[11] Evers et al. in 1991 studied the cumulative literature data from studies reporting recurrent endometriosis and showed that there is gradual but steady increase in the incidence of recurrence over a period of 5 years follow-up.

## Site of Recurrence

In 2005, Vignali M et al.[7] published a follow-up study among symptomatic patients who were operated for deep infiltrating endometriosis (DIE) with postoperative follow-up for at least 12 months, analysis revealed that age, obliteration of pouch of Douglas (POD) and surgical completeness may play significant role in the recurrence of the disease. During follow-up and analysis, approximately. 20.5% and 9% showed recurrence of pain and clinical findings, respectively.

Exacoustos et al.[11] (2006) reported recurrence occurred in the same ovary in 81% of patients, 11% showed recurrence of lesion in the contralateral untreated ovary and 8% showed involvement of both ovaries. 20% of patients showed recurrence after 1st surgical procedure and 17% after 2nd procedure at the end of 5 years.[12]

## DIAGNOSIS OF RECURRENCE

Diagnosis is influenced by reappearance of symptoms, clinical examination, USG evidence of endometriosis, biomarker (which characterize the progress of disease), laparoscopy and presence of biopsy proven endometriosis. Imaging modalities like USG and MRI pick up the recurrent lesions, but their extent cannot be made out [European Society of Human Reproduction and Embryology (ESHRE) guidelines level A evidence]. Pelvic pain and dyspareunia are the common symptoms of recurrence following hysterectomy. Sometimes vaginal and rectal bleeding, low backache, and rectal pain may occur. Chapron et al. 2005 reported dyschezia and severe dyspareunia indicating deeply infiltrating lesions. As the differential diagnosis is broad, the exact cause of pain may be difficult to isolate.

## ROLE OF BIOMARKERS

In endometriotic patients, the role of biomarkers is not specific, but it can provide information regarding disease progression and treatment effectiveness. Molecular and genetic differences intrinsic to lesion may confer different risks of endometriosis recurrence. Cyclooxygenase-2 (COX-2) overexpression, previous medical management, presence of adhesions are few predictors of recurrence. Rapid advances in genomics, epigenomics, and proteomics may pave way for newer biomarkers.

ER$\alpha$ and ER$\beta$ are two forms of estrogen receptors, which show an E-binding domain and DNA-binding domain, respectively. *ER$\alpha$* gene polymorphism is more associated with recurrence if P-vull *ER$\alpha$* gene homozygosity is detected (Luisi et al.).[13]

Cyclooxygenase-2 being a rate-limiting enzyme of prostaglandin synthesis is actively involved in inflammation and proliferation of endometriotic lesions. The concentration of prostaglandins are increased in the peritoneal fluid of infertile women with endometriosis.

Nuclear factor-kappa B (NF-kB) promotes expression of more than 150 genes in cellular processors. Along with p50, p52, p65, c-Rel and Rel-B, NF-kB is involved in DNA binding and regulation. These markers are detected in high-risk patients with recurrence.[14,15]

In 2008, Yuan et al.[16] and Liu et al. 2007[13] showed a prediction of recurrence with 30 months of surgery with sensitivity and specificity of 72%. In endometriotic tissue recovered at surgery, there is decreasing progesterone receptor (PR)-B receptor activity, increased COX-2 expression, increased NF-kB activation, claudin 3, claudin 4, heparanase-1 and phosphatase of regenerating liver-3. Previously treated patients (medically) and presence of adhesions are risk factors for recurrence.[16]

Biomarkers till date are used only for research purposes (ESHRE guidelines level A evidence).

## TREATMENT OF RECURRENT ENDOMETRIOSIS

Laparoscopy is the gold standard in diagnosis as well as treatment of recurrent endometriosis. Three goals of the treatment include delaying recurrence, reducing pain and treating infertility.[17] Therefore, the main aim is providing complete cure (which is not possible).

## PREVENTING RECURRENCE

Recurrence of endometriotic lesion can be avoided by ablating all endometriotic lesions. However, smaller atypical lesions are overlooked leading to disease persistence.

## TIMING OF SURGERY

Since 1980, laparoscopy has revolutionized the treatment, and surgery must be done during the follicular phase. Techniques such as excision, coagulation, vaporization of lesions, and laser may delay the recurrence. Patients who had surgery in luteal phase showed short remissions and had two-fold increase in recurrence rate 1 year later.

## TECHNIQUE OF SURGERY

Ultrasonography or laparoscopic-guided drainage of endometriomas has 80–100% recurrence within 6 months, whereas cyst drainage with cyst wall destruction showed 3 times more recurrence than cystectomy (18.4 vs. 6.4). Cystectomy is considered superior to drainage and coagulation in ovarian endometrioma (>3 cm). In DIE, resection of rectovaginal nodule relieves pain rapidly. Radical surgery is often mandatory in preventing recurrence, in patients who have completed family[18] **(Fig. 1)**. There should be a balance when performing surgery for endometrioma as too little is going to cause recurrence and too much is going to cost impaired ovarian reserve.

## PROTECTIVE FACTORS

Pregnancy, oral contraceptive pill (OCP) usage, postoperative progestin use and gonadotropin-releasing hormone (GnRH) analogs (as adjuvant therapy) are few factors which postpone the recurrence of endometriosis.[6]

### Preoperative Medical Management

Preoperative medical management alone may increase the risk of recurrence if no postoperative treatment is provided. Medications might mask some

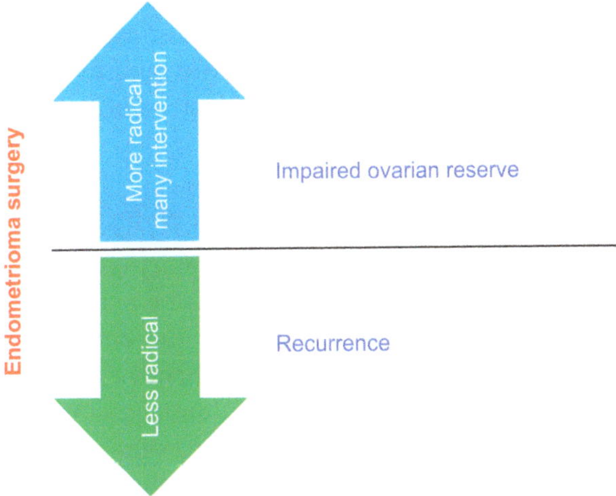


**Fig. 1:** Endometrioma surgery.

lesions during surgery making them difficult to resect. Lesions may recur if medications are discontinued abruptly.

## Postoperative Medication and Recurrence Risk

Postoperative medical treatment should be administrated to minimize the risk of recurrence and extend pain-free period in severe disease after conservative surgery.

The main focus is eliminating the residual endometriotic cells.[6] Some patients show progestin resistance and downregulation of PR-B receptors, so combination of drugs in a trial and error fashion should be given targeting reduction in recurrence. The effect of drugs given postoperatively vanishes soon after stopping the drugs. Hence, it is only for temporary protection. Long-term OCPs, dienogest, GnRH analogs, and levonorgestrel-releasing intrauterine system (LNG-IUS) are best in preventing recurrence and can be given for women not desirous of pregnancy (ESHRE Guidelines, 2014).

### Role of Nonsteroidal Anti-inflammatory Drugs

Cochrane review states that nonsteroidal anti-inflammatory drugs (NSAIDs) provide only symptomatic pain management. They are ineffective in curing the disease.[19]

### Role of Oral Contraceptive Pills

Oral contraceptive pills act by ovarian suppression, decreasing retrograde menstruation and by inhibiting proliferation of endometriosis, thus, aids in reducing pain and recurrence rates. Continuous OCP administration is far better than intermittent therapy. The recurrence rate is reduced by end of 1 year but not at the end of 2–3 years (similar to placebo)**(Fig. 2)**.[6,10]

Seracchioli et al.[20] showed that continuous or cyclical usage of OCPs provided significant results among patients who reported with recurrence. Continuous OCPs usage might be preferred instead of cyclical treatment if the latter fails to provide pain relief.[21]

### Levonorgestrel-releasing Intrauterine System in Recurrence Prevention

Through its anti-inflammatory, immunomodulatory effect, downregulating the proliferative endometrial cells and by causing endometrial glandular atrophy, LNG-IUS reduced dysmenorrhea at the end of 1 year by 10% as against 45% in nonusers. LNG-IUS is as effective as GnRH analogs.[22] Vercellini et al.[22] in 2003 conducted a randomized controlled trial and reported that postsurgical use of LNG-IUS reduces the recurrence risk after 1 year when compared with patients who were only observed after surgery for endometriosis.

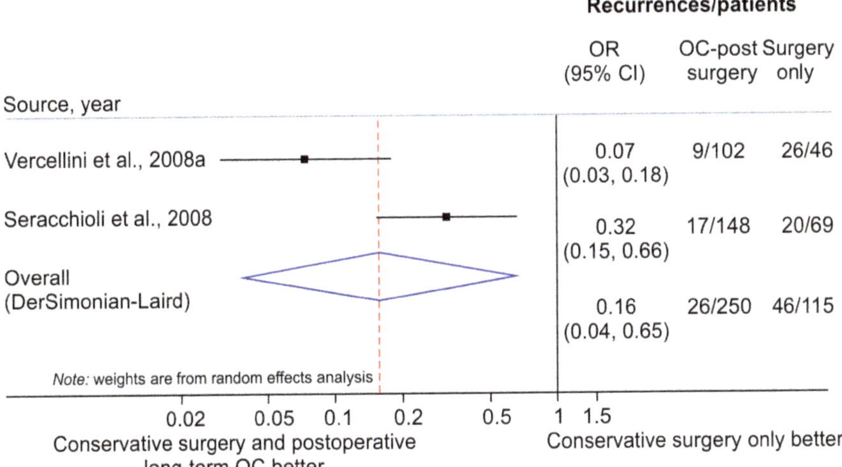



**Fig. 2:** Meta-analysis performed to know the variation in recurrence of endometriosis between conservative surgery and conservative surgery followed by long-term COCs. This depicts that only conservative surgery is inferior to conservative surgery followed by long term COCs.

## *Postoperative GnRH Analogs' Role in Preventing Recurrence*

Gonadotropin-releasing hormone analogs reduce inflammation and adhesions when given postoperatively for 6 months. Patients showed a drastic response to pain at the end of 12-month and 24-month follow-up. Unfortunately, GnRH analogs did not reduce the recurrence in stage III and IV; instead, it delayed the time of recurrence.[2] Unfortunately, the recurrence rate at the end of 5 years were similar to placebo users (53.4%).

## *Danazol*

Telimaa et al. proposed that medroxyprogesterone acetate (MPA) and danazol, when used postoperatively, reduced the pain scores. But, the results were more valuable when used for at least 6 months.

Morgante et al.[2] reported that postoperative administration of low-dose danazol (100 mg/day for 6 months) reduced pelvic pain when compared with nonusers. Despite this, Bianchi et al. concluded that there is no role of danazol on postoperative recurrence rate (when 600 mg/day was given for 3 months). A ratio of 26% and 34% were reported between one group on danazol and the other group who were not on danazol.[23] This study showed that there was no difference in recurrence rate between the two groups.

## *Tibolone*

Tibolone causes atrophy of endometrial tissue theoretically exhibiting similar effects on ectopic endometrial tissue as well (Soliman and Hilliard, 2006).

A randomized trial among 21 women with residual pelvic endometriosis after bilateral oophorectomy who were on tibolone (n = 11) are transdermal estrogen with medroxyprogesterone acetate (n = 12) were followed up for 12 months. Fedele et al. 1999 reported that only one patient (9%) from the tibolone group reported symptomatic recurrence, compared with 4 (40%) in the combined hormone replacement therapy (HRT) group.

With all the above treatment options, it is important to individualize the plan of management according to the patient characteristics, side effect profile and the individual's choice by thorough counseling and actively involving the woman in the choice of treatment.

## MEDICAL MANAGEMENT IN RECURRENCE PREVENTION

Management mainly focuses on pain relief either medically or surgically. Drugs like danazol, and GnRH are restricted to 6 months use only due to the side effects (beyond 6 months usage needs add-back therapy) whereas OCPs, and progestins can be given for longer durations. Depot MPA, dienogest, cabergoline, aromatase inhibitors, and LNG-IUS are other options available. However, selection of choice of treatment has to be done carefully. In infertile women, repeat surgery has to be restricted as it affects ovarian reserve (ESHRE Guidelines, 2014).

## SURGICAL MANAGEMENT OF PAIN

Surgery is superior to medical management to treat pain recurrence as the effect of drugs is short lived and are more expensive. Laparoscopy can excise all the lesions, thereby restoring the pelvic anatomy. Ureteric dissection has to be carefully done to prevent complications.

Surgery with long-term suppression using drugs has to be considered in recurrent endometrioma and pain management. Definite surgery must be chosen based on patient's requirement. Conservative surgery is indicated in patients who are desirous of retaining the uterus and the ovaries. Here they can be offered ablation or excision of the implants, cystectomy in case of endometrioma and adhesiolysis to regain the pelvic anatomy. Laparoscopic uterine nerve ablation is not effective for pain management. Presacral neurectomy is effective but can lead to newer long-term problems (ESHRE Guidelines, 2014). In patients who have completed the family, they can be advised hysterectomy with/without bilateral salphingo oophorectomy and excision of the peritoneal lesions. There is always a higher risk of recurrence and necessity for redo surgeries if ovaries are left behind **(Table 3)**.

### Presacral Neurectomy (Pelvic Denervation)

Presacral neurectomy (PSN) effectively reduces pain recurrence, particularly midline pain, whereas lateral and adnexal pain is not relieved. PSN

**Table 3:** Recurrence rates in surgeries with and without uterosacral resection.

| Conservative | Definitive |
| --- | --- |
| Ablation/excision of implants | Bilateral salphingo-oophorectomy (BSO) |
| Cystectomy/ablation of endometriotic cysts | Hysterectomy |
| Adhesiolysis | Hysterectomy plus BSO |
| Ureter mobilization | All the above plus implant excision |
| Laparoscopic uterine nerve ablation | |
| Presacral nerve ablation | |

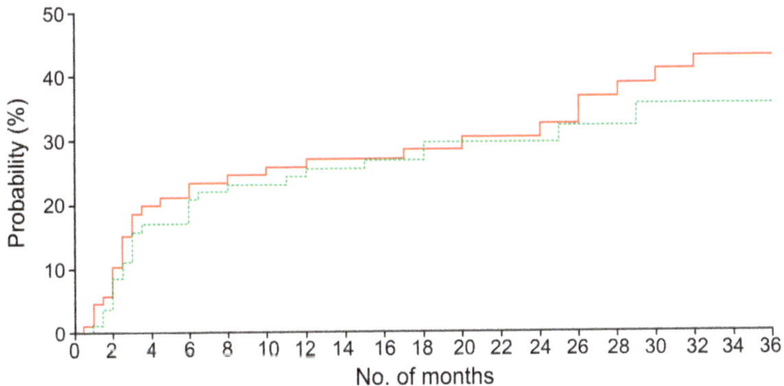

**Fig. 3:** Cumulative 36-month probability recurrence of moderate or severe dysmenorrhea, as assessed by a linear analogue scale in 180 symptomatic women with endometriosis who had laparoscopic surgery with (solid line) or without (dashed line) uterosacral ligament resection.

effectiveness is based on surgeon's experience. Denervation of bowel and bladder leads to constipation and urinary dysfunction.[24,25]

According to a Cochrane meta-analysis, the addition of laparoscopic uterine nerve ablation (LUNA) to laparoscopic surgical treatment of endometriosis did not give relief from secondary dysmenorrhea [Odds ratio (OR) 0.77], whereas PSN did (OR 3.14). ESHRE guidelines are also in favor of the same **(Fig. 3)**.

Busacca et al.[26] published an article demonstrating whether laparotomy versus laparoscopy is effective in surgical treatment of recurrent endometriosis. It depends upon the skill of the surgeon.

Deep endometriotic lesions in subperitoneal space may be difficult to visualize laparoscopically. Also, lesions can be hidden by peritoneal adhesion of POD. Such microscopic foci could progress under favorable conditions clinically paving way to disease recurrence. Patients who underwent hysterectomy with ovarian preservation had 6 times more chance for pain recurrence and 8 times greater risk of reoperation.[27]

| Summary recommendations ASRM/ESHRE | |
| --- | --- |
| Asymptomatic women with endometriosis, surgical treatment guidelines: | |
| **Clinical condition** | **Recommendation** |
| Stage I-II | Limited benefit: Surgery recommended |
| Stage III-IV | Possible but unproven benefit: Surgery recommended |
| Postoperative adjuvant treatment | No benefit: Not recommended |
| Surgery before IVF | Doubtful benefit: Perhaps for endometrioma ≥4 cm |
| Recurrent endometriosis | Not recommended |

**Fig. 4:** Surgical treatment guidelines for asymptomatic women with endometriosis.

Ovarian preservation is essential as many endometriotic patients undergoing hysterectomy are young women in whom to preserving at least one ovary has to be considered.

## INFERTILITY MANAGEMENT IN RECURRENCE

Surgery has to be meticulous in infertile women. There is approximately 50% reduction in fertility following repeat surgery. Ovarian endometriomas <3 cm can be conservatively managed. Assisted reproductive technology (ART) is recommended to patients desirous of pregnancy. Surgery is indicated in the presence of pain, difficulty in oocyte pick up and malignancy suspicion. Repeat surgery for infertility is associated with lower pregnancy rates due to reduced ovarian reserve. According to ASRM and ESHRE guidelines, IVF is preferred over surgery in patients with recurrence with infertility and all the more when there is no pain or risk of malignancy. In vitro fertilization (IVF) is preferred over surgery in patients with infertility, when there is no pain and risk of malignancy (ESHRE Guidelines, 2014) **(Fig. 4)**.

## HORMONAL REPLACEMENT THERAPY AFTER SURGERY FOR ENDOMETRIOSIS

Initiation of HRT following hysterectomy in endometriotic patients is not recommended clearly. Most recent guidelines suggests that HRT is not contraindicated. Bulletin in 2010 [American College of Obstetricians and Gynecologists (ACOG)]:

Accurate incidence of recurrence with HRT is unknown. A prospective randomized study (follow-up interval was 45 months) by Matorras et al. in 2002 estimating the risk of recurrence associated with combined HRT (n = 115) versus nonusers (n = 57) among patients who underwent bilateral salphingo-oopherectomy with or without hysterectomy (91.8% underwent hysterectomy) for endometriosis. The recurrence rate were 3.5% in women under HRT (4 in 115) and 0.9% per year. Two patients were reoperated. Women who were not on HRT had no recurrence. Peritoneal involvement more than 3% (with 2.4% recurrence per year vs. 0.3%) and incomplete surgery (22.2% per year vs. 1.9%) were the two major risk factors associated with recurrence in women who received HRT. The author concluded that additional care is mandatory in patients with peritoneal involvement, though the risk of recurrence is low.

## CONCLUSION

Clinically, it is difficult to totally eliminate the risk of recurrence after treating endometriosis. Though literature offers a variety of risk factors, it is always convenient to group them based on the patients' necessity (with or without infertility treatment). Use of OCPs diminishes the risk of recurrence after surgery when administered for longer duration. An ideal biomarker for recurrence should be identified which will help in understanding the pathophysiology and reduce the risk of factors related with the disease. COX-2 and NF-kB are two important biomarkers of recurrence. However, only limited studies are available focusing on the recurrence of endometriosis.

## REFERENCES


1. Busacca M, Marana R, Caruana P, Candiani M, Muzii L, Calia C, et al. Recurrence of ovarian endometrioma after laparoscopic excision. Am J Obstet Gynecol. 1999;180(3):519-23.
2. Morgante G, Ditto A, La Marca A, De Leo V. Low-dose danazol after combined surgical and medical therapy reduces the incidence of pelvic pain in women with moderate and severe endometriosis. Hum Reprod. 1999;14(9):2371-4.
3. Busacca M, Chiaffarino F, Candiani M, Vignali M, Bertulessi C, Oggioni G, et al. Determinants of long-term clinically detected recurrence rates of deep, ovarian, and pelvic endometriosis. Am J Obstet Gynecol. 2006;195(2):426-32.
4. Ghezzi F, Beretta P, Franchi M, Parissis M, Bolis P. Recurrence of ovarian endometriosis and anatomical location of the primary lesion. Fertil Steril. 2001;75(1):136-40.
5. Parazzini F, Bertulessi C, Pasini A, Rosati M, Di Stefano F, Shonauer S, et al. Determinants of short term recurrence rate of endometriosis. Eur J Obstet Gynecol Reprod Biol. 2005;121(2):216-9.
6. Guo SW. Recurrence of endometriosis and its control. Human reproduction update. 2009;15(4):441-61.
7. Vignali M, Bianchi S, Candiani M, Spadaccini G, Oggioni G, Busacca M. Surgical treatment of deep endometriosis and risk of recurrence. J Minim Invasive Gynecol. 2005;12(6):508-13.
8. Barrier BF, Dick EJ Jr, Butler SD, Hubbard GB. Endometriosis involving the ileocaecal junction with regional lymph node involvement in the baboon—striking pathological finding identical between the human and the baboon: a case report. Hum Reprod. 2006;22(1):272-4.
9. Maeda N, Izumiya C, Kusum T, Masumoto T, Yamashita C, Yamamoto Y, et al. Killer inhibitory receptor CD158a overexpression among natural killer cells in women with

endometriosis is undiminished by laparoscopic surgery and gonadotropin releasing hormone agonist treatment. Am J Reprod Immunol. 2004;51(5):364-72.

10. Selçuk İ, Bozdağ G. Recurrence of endometriosis; risk factors, mechanisms and biomarkers; review of the literature. J Turk Ger Gynecol Assoc. 2013;14(2):98.

11. Exacoustos C, Zupi E, Amadio A, Amoroso C, Szabolcs B, Romanini ME, et al. Recurrence of endometriomas after laparoscopic removal: sonographic and clinical follow-up and indication for second surgery. J Minim Invasive Gynecol. 2006;13(4):281-8.

12. Fedele L, Bianchi S, Zanconato G, Berlanda N, Raffaelli R, Fontana E. Laparoscopic excision of recurrent endometriomas: long-term outcome and comparison with primary surgery. Fertil Steril. 2006;85(3):694-9.

13. Luisi S, Galleri L, Marini F, Ambrosini G, Brandi ML, Petraglia F. Estrogen receptor gene polymorphisms are associated with recurrence of endometriosis. Fertil Steril. 2006;85(3):764-6.

14. Kumar A, Takada Y, Boriek AM, Aggarwal BB. Nuclear factor-kappaB: its role in health and disease. J Mol Med (Berl). 2004;82(7):434-48.

15. Guo SW. Nuclear factor-kappaB (NF-kappaB): an unsuspected major culprit in the pathogenesis of endometriosis that is still at large? Gynecol Obstet Invest. 2007;63(2):71-97.

16. Yuan L, Shen F, Lu Y, Liu X, Guo SW. Cyclooxygenase-2 overexpression in ovarian endometriomas is associated with higher risk of recurrence. Fertil Steril. 2009;91(4):1303-6.

17. Donnez J, Pirard C, Smets M, Jadoul P, Squifflet J. Surgical management of endometriosis. Best Pract Res Clin Obstet Gynaecol. 2004;18(2):329-48.

18. Sesti F, Capozzolo T, Pietropolli A, Marziali M, Bollea MR, Piccione E. Recurrence rate of endometrioma after laparoscopic cystectomy: a comparative randomized trial between post-operative hormonal suppression treatment or dietary therapy vs. placebo. Eur J Obstet Gynecol Reprod Biol. 2009;147(1):72-7.

19. Allen C, Hopewell S, Prentice A, Gregory D. Nonsteroidal anti-inflammatory drugs for pain in women with endometriosis. Cochrane Database Syst Rev. 2009;(2):CD004753.

20. Seracchioli R, Mabrouk M, Frasca C, Manuzzi L, Montanari G, Keramyda A, et al. Long-term cyclic and continuous oral contraceptive therapy and endometrioma recurrence: a randomized controlled trial. Fertil Steril. 2010;93(1):52-6.

21. Vercellini P, Frontino G, De Giorgi O, Pietropaolo G, Pasin R, Crosignani PG. Continuous use of an oral contraceptive for endometriosis-associated recurrent dysmenorrhea that does not respond to a cyclic pill regimen. Fertil Steril. 2003;80(3):560-3.

22. Vercellini P, Frontino G, De Giorgi O, Aimi G, Zaina B, Crosignani PG. Comparison of a levonorgestrel-releasing intrauterine device versus expectant management after conservative surgery for symptomatic endometriosis: a pilot study. Fertil Steril. 2003;80(2):305-9.

23. Bianchi S, Busacca M, Agnoli B, Candiani M, Calia C, Vignali M. Effects of 3 month therapy with danazol after laparoscopic surgery for stage III/IV endometriosis: a randomized study. Hum Reprod. 1999;14(5):1335-7.

24. Zullo F, Palomba S, Zupi E, Russo T, Morelli M, Sena T, et al. Long-term effectiveness of presacral neurectomy for the treatment of severe dysmenorrhea due to endometriosis. J Am Assoc Gynecol Laparosc. 2004;11(1):23-8.

25. Vercellini P, Barbara G, Abbiati A, Somigliana E, Viganò P, Fedele L. Repetitive surgery for recurrent symptomatic endometriosis: what to do?. Eur J Obstet Gynecol Reprod Biol. 2009;146(1):15-21.

26. Busacca M, Fedele L, Bianchi S, Candiani M, Agnoli B, Raffaelli R, et al. Surgical treatment of recurrent endometriosis: laparotomy versus laparoscopy. Hum Reprod. 1998;13(8):2271-4.

27. Rizk B, Fischer AS, Lotfy HA, Turki R, Zahed HA, Malik R, et al. Recurrence of endometriosis after hysterectomy. Facts Views Vis Obgyn. 2014;6(4):219.

# CHAPTER 8

# Infertility Associated with Endometriosis

*Kanthi Bansal*

## INTRODUCTION

Endometriosis is a mysterious disease and the two important impacts are pain and infertility. Till date, the exact etiology of infertility in cases of endometriosis is not clear but multiple factors are involved. The causative factors also include adhesions and disturbed endocrine factors. There is distortion of the anatomy, the oocyte is affected, tubal dysfunction is there, and the immune system is disturbed in many cases of unexplained infertility. As the disease is complex, the diagnosis is difficult. The management of infertility is assisted reproductive techniques (ART); conservative treatment has minimal role.

## ETIOLOGY OF INFERTILITY ASSOCIATED WITH ENDOMETRIOSIS

In infertile women, the presence of mild endometriosis is frequent; however, the severity of disease and grade of endometriosis is the reason for infertility. With expectant management, 40% mild-grade patients conceive, whereas very few patients with moderate-to-severe endometriosis are successful.[1]

It is not yet clear about the mechanism of endometriosis-related infertility but is different in different stages of endometriosis:

- *Distortion of anatomy*: Due to the endometriosis implants in the pelvic region, the anatomy is distorted. There is hindrance to the transport of oocyte and/or embryo to the endometrial cavity. There are additions which could be one of the causes of restricted mobility of the fimbrial end of the fallopian tube.[2]
- *Altered peritoneal function*:[3,4] Alterations in peritoneal fluid impact sperm, oocyte, embryo, or fallopian tube function.[5-7]
- *Hormonal change and cell-mediated function*: Immunoglobulin A (IgA) and IgG autoantibodies and lymphocytes alter implantation and receptivity of endometrium. Autoantibodies to endometrial antigens can increase endocrine and ovulatory abnormalities.[7-12]
- *Implantation and endometrial receptivity*: Inflammation of peritoneum affects the implantation rates and receptivity of endometrium. This is due to the increase in activity of macrophages and cell molecule adhesions. More recently, very low levels of an enzyme involved in the synthesis of

the endometrial ligand for L-selectin (a protein that coats the trophoblast on the surface of the blastocyst) have been observed in infertile women with endometriosis.

The endometrial receptivity is inadequately expressed due to decrease in expression of biomarkers of implantation, such as glycodelin A, osteopontin, lysophosphatidic acid receptor 3, and HOXA10 and integrins (cell adhesion molecule) in the women with endometriosis. This shows that the endometrial receptivity in patients with endometriosis is damaged. Also, this increases the chances of ectopic pregnancies.[13-15]

- *Quality of oocytes and embryos*: The production of oocyte and the process of ovulation are affected due to endometriomas. The affected ovary is also associated with the increased inflammatory cells in the peritoneal fluid and a luteal phase disruption.[16]
- *Uterotubal transport*: The tubal function is affected due to inflammation and it also impairs the tubal motility. Transport of gamete and implantation of embryos are also affected due to abnormal myometrial contractions associated with endometriosis.

## ENDOMETRIOSIS FERTILITY INDEX

The endometriosis fertility index (EFI) is used to predict fecundity after endometriosis surgery. In addition to providing a detailed score to the appendix (fallopian tubes, fimbriae of fallopian tubes, and ovaries) by calculating the least-function scores, the EFI also combines conception-related factors such as age, duration of infertility, and gravidity history. The EFI score ranges from 0 to 10 (0—poorest prognosis, 10—best prognosis).[17]

| Structure | Dysfunction | Description |
| --- | --- | --- |
| Tube | Mild | Slight injury to serosa of the fallopian tube |
| | Moderate | Moderate injury to serosa or muscularis of the fallopian tube; moderate limitation in mobility |
| | Severe | Fallopian tube fibrosis or mild/moderate salpingitis isthmica nodosa; severe limitation in mobility |
| | Nonfunctional | Complete tubal obstruction, extensive fibrosis, or salpingitis isthmica nodosa |
| Fimbria | Mild | Slight injury to fimbria with minimal scarring |
| | Moderate | Moderate injury to fimbria, with moderate scarring, moderate loss of fimbrial Architecture, and minimal intrafimbrial fibrosis |
| | Severe | Severe injury fimbria, with severe scarring, severe loss of fimbrial architecture, and moderate intrafimbrial fibrosis |
| | Nonfunctional | Severe injury to fimbria, with extensive scarring, complete loss of fimbrial architecture, complete tubal occlusion, or hydrosalpinx |

*Contd...*

*Contd...*

| Structure | Dysfunction | Description |
|---|---|---|
| Ovary | Mild | Normal or almost normal ovarian size; minimal or mild injury to ovarian serosa |
| | Moderate | Ovarian size reduced by one-third or more; moderate injury to ovarian surface |
| | Severe | Ovarian size reduced by two-thirds or more; severe injury to ovarian surface |
| | Nonfunctional | Ovary absent or completely encased in adhesions[18] |

## MANAGEMENT OF INFERTILITY ASSOCIATED WITH ENDOMETRIOSIS

### Medical Management

The patients with endometriosis are advised hormonal therapies but they have contraceptive effects. A meta-analysis was done by Hughes et al.[19]on whether the hormonal treatment has any role in the infertility treatment caused by endometriosis. The study showed that suppression of ovarian function in minimal-to-mild endometriosis by danazol, gonadotropin-releasing hormone (GnRH) analogs, or oral contraceptive pills (OCPs) is not effective and should not be offered for this indication alone.[20] According to Cochrane review, there is no difference between different drugs and their effects on spontaneous pregnancy or live birth rates when compared to placebo or no treatment.[19] Hence, patients who wish to conceive cannot be advised hormonal ovarian suppression to treat infertility as the first line of treatment.

The fourth-generation progestin of 19-nortestosterone derivative, dienogest, is the only medical option. It is well tolerated with no androgenic, glucocorticoid, or mineralocorticoid activity, binds to the progesterone receptor with high specificity, and produces a potent progestogenic effect related to the high circulating levels of the unbound molecule. Dienogest is associated with relatively moderate inhibition of gonadotropin secretion, leading to a reduction in the endogenous production of estradiol. When given continuously, dienogest induces a hypoestrogenic, local endocrine environment causing a decidualization of endometrial tissue followed by atrophy of the endometriotic lesions. It also inhibits aromatase and cyclooxygenase-2 (COX-2) expression as well as prostaglandin E2 production in endometriotic stromal cells. It also normalizes the activity of natural killer cells and decreases the release of interleukin-1b by macrophages. Dienogest increases progesterone receptor expression and decreases proinflammatory cytokines.

The optimal dose is 2 mg once daily in the treatment of endometriosis for duration of 12–24 weeks. Several trials are going on to assess the role of dienogest pretreatment for endometriosis in comparison to GnRH agonist in patients of endometriosis undergoing in vitro fertilization (IVF) with hypothetical results, no significant difference was noted in the number of oocyte retrieved, pregnancy, and miscarriage rate. Further studies and trials for validation of these results are still needed.[21,22]

> **Recommendation—GCPR on Endometriosis-FOGSI:**
> - Medical management in the form of ovulation suppression is ineffective in improving the pregnancy rates (Evidence level A).[23,24]
> - Guideline Development Group (GDG) recommends no benefits of adjunctive hormonal therapy before surgery to improve spontaneous pregnancy rates (Evidence level GPP).
> - Clinicians should not prescribe adjunctive hormonal therapy after surgery to improve spontaneous pregnancy rates (Evidence level A).[25]
> - GDG does not recommend nutritional supplement, complementary or alternate medicine in the treatment of endometriosis-associated infertility (Evidence level GPP).[26]

> **Recommendation—GCPR on Endometriosis-FOGSI:**
> - Ultra-long protocol of GnRH agonists for a period of 3–6 months before ART improves the clinical pregnancy rates (Evidence level A).

## Surgical Management

### *Preoperative Medical Management: Not Recommended*

- Changes in the appearance of endometriosis
- Delay of diagnosis
- Cost and side effects
- Delay attempting pregnancy
- No difference for pain relief or infertility.

### *Postoperative Medical Management: No Evidence of Benefit*

Women with endometriosis should not be prescribed adjunctive hormonal treatment after surgery to improve spontaneous pregnancy rates.

Laparoscopy is the gold standard for the endometriosis. Surgical treatment is more efficient by ablating the lesions for the improvement of fertility in the type of minimal-to-mild endometriosis and pain relief is advantage.[27]

Laparoscopic cystectomy is better when compared to drainage and coagulation in endometrioma.[28] For recurrence endometrioma, more positive outcome is achieved by excision with regard to the recurrence of pain symptoms, and in women who were previously subfertile, subsequent pregnancy occurs. Both the Cochrane reviews and the Royal College of Obstetricians and Gynaecologists (RCOG) guidelines are in agreement that there is definite improvement in fertility associated with endometriosis following laparoscopic surgery.[13] Cochrane review suggests that excision cystectomy is the ideal method for endometrial cysts in pain and fertility and

**Table 1:** International guidelines for surgical treatment of endometriosis-associated infertility in asymptomatic women.[18]

| Clinical condition | ESHRE 2014 | ASRM 2012 | RCOG 2006 |
|---|---|---|---|
| Minimal–mild (stage I–II) | Demonstrated benefit: surgery recommended | Small benefit: insufficient to recommend surgery solely to increase the likelihood of pregnancy | Demonstrated benefit: surgery recommended |
| Moderate–severe (stage III–IV) | Possible benefit: surgery can be considered | Possible benefit: surgery may be beneficial | Possible benefit: recommendation uncertain |
| Postoperative adjuvant treatment | No benefit: not recommended | No benefit: not recommended | No benefit: not recommended |
| Surgery before IVF | Uncertain benefit in stage I–II: may be considered. No benefit if endo-metrioma >3 cm: only considered to improve pain or the accessibility of follicles | Insufficient benefit: no recommendation surgery should be considered if endo-metrioma >4 cm | Recommended if endometrioma >4 cm |
| Recurrent endometriosis | Surgery should be considered carefully if the women has had previous ovarian surgery | Second-line surgery not recommended; IVF-ET is an effective alternative | No recommenda-tion |

(ASRM: American Society for Reproductive Medicine; ESHRE: European Society of Human Reproduction and Embryology; ET: embryo transfer; IVF: in vitro fertilization; RCOG: Royal College of Obstetricians and Gynaecologists)

can be aided by the use of Mesna and initial circular excision. An absorbable adhesion barrier, 4% icodextrin solution, and a viscoelastic gel are safe and beneficial products for reducing the adhesion formation in laparoscopic surgery.

Excision technique is related to increase in the rate of pregnancy and a decrease in the rate of recurrence can lead to severe damage to the ovarian reserve as per randomized controlled trials (RCTs).[29,30] Combined excision-vaporization technique or replacement of diathermy coagulation by suture may improve the latter aspect **(Table 1)**.[31]

Recommendation—GCPR on Endometriosis FOGSI:
- Laparoscopic ablation or excision and adhesiolysis improve pregnancy rate in stages I and II endometriosis when compared to diagnostic laparoscopy alone (Evidence level A).[32,33]

*Contd...*

*Contd...*

- Operative laparoscopy is the treatment for stages III and IV endometriosis to increase spontaneous pregnancy rate (Evidence level B).[34]
- Excision of endometrioma, i.e., cystectomy is better than drainage or coagulation and is recommended as the treatment of choice (Evidence level A).[34,35]
- The GDG recommends clinicians to counsel women with endometrioma regarding the reduction of ovarian reserve following surgery. In the event of previous surgery, the decisions for repeat surgery should be done carefully (Evidence level GPP).
- Excision of endometrioma is strongly recommended in infertile women, when there is suspicion of malignancy or when there is rupture or torsion of the cyst (Evidence level A).[26]

## GNRH AGONIST FOR THE INFERTILITY TREATMENT IN ENDOMETRIOSIS

One of the hypotheses says that GnRH agonist acts by regulating the mechanisms of apoptosis and angiogenesis on cells of endometrium and thus inhibiting their growth and proliferation.

There are some latest studies which show that GnRH agonist decreases vascular endothelial growth factor A (VEGF-A) and IL-1β production in the endometrium cells and inhibiting the increases in endometriosis. Randomized studies suggest that GnRH agonist to be given for 3–6 months but Cochrane review called for further research. The course of treatment is 3–6 months but treatment for 6 months appears to lead to a longer delay before the return of symptoms.[36,37]

The rate of recurrence of endometriosis is directly proportional to duration and grade of disease. After surgery, GnRH agonist for 6 months may decrease the pain for 12–24 months when compared to expectant management or placebo. Treatment with GnRH agonists for 6 months had a beneficial impact on ultrasonographic recurrence rate after conservative laparoscopic surgery for ovarian endometriosis (endometriosis stage III/IV) at 24/36-month follow-up.[38]

## OVARIAN ENDOMETRIOMA

There is still controversy in understanding the role of endometrioma in leading to infertility but a study showed that patients with infertility due to endometriosis present 17–44% ovarian endometrioma. A large endometrioma may replace most of the normal ovarian tissue. Presence of peritubal and periovarian adhesions may distort the pelvic anatomy. Follicular defects such as abnormal follicular growth, decreased follicular size, and shortened follicular phase are observed in women with mild endometriosis. Impaired ovarian function, pituitary ovarian dysfunction, granulosa cell impairment, and uterine function impact on oocyte quality and embryo quality, resulting in ovulatory, fertilization, and implantation disorders.[39]

In endometrioma, the follicular development is compromised and the quality of oocyte and embryos is poor, which lead to decrease in fertility outcomes. Surgical removal of endometrioma leads to decline in ovarian reserve and the response to stimulation. Expectant management, aspiration with ultrasonography (USG), endometriotic cyst drainage and vaporization of the cyst wall, ovarian fenestration with bipolar electrocoagulation, and laparoscopic cystectomy are advised for endometrioma with infertility. Regarding spontaneous pregnancies and recurrence of the cysts and symptoms, a recent systemic review shows that laparoscopic cystectomy is the best treatment compared to drainage or coagulation.[40]

Alborzi et al. prospectively evaluated 52 patients submitted to laparoscopic cystectomy and observed spontaneous pregnancy rates of nearly 60% in the first year after surgery, which were statistically significant when compared with the 23.3% obtained after endometrioma fenestration and coagulation.[41]

After surgery, for patients under 35 years of age, expectant therapy can be a good choice for spontaneous pregnancy, but patients over 35 years of age or patients with ovarian functional impairment should not go for expectant treatment as they have low ovarian reserve and low ovarian response. For such patient, ART has to be considered as the first line of treatment.[38]

For ovarian endometrioma ≥4 cm in diameter, laparoscopic ovarian cystectomy is suggested. Surgical approach confirms the diagnosis as histological examination can be performed, reduces the risk of recurrence, better access to follicles, increased ovarian response, and prevents endometriosis progression. There is risk of reduced ovarian function postsurgery for which a woman needs to be counseled[42,43] and the decision should be reconsidered if she has had previous ovarian surgery.[29] Garcia-Velasco et al. has done a retrospective study where 189 women who had undergone IVF treatment were evaluated following laparoscopic approach to excise lesions and observed no differences between the groups, whatever variety analyzed. The study found 25.4% of pregnancies among operated women and 22.7% among patients with intact cysts, with no statistical significance, and concluded that no additional benefits were provided by cystectomy.[42]

Normal ovarian tissue removal might have a negative effect on controlled ovarian hyperstimulation (COH) due to cystectomy.[43]

Accidental removal of ovarian tissue during cystectomy and the damage inflicted by both surgery-related local inflammation and electrosurgical coagulation of ovarian stroma and vascularization may add to the problem but do not affect the mean number of dominant follicles and pregnancy rate.

## TREATMENT OF ENDOMETRIOMA BEFORE STARTING IN VITRO FERTILIZATION

Commonly, in clinical practice, it is found that many patients who are planning for ART have endometrioma. Ovarian reserve is reduced due to surgical excision and there is reduction in healthy tissue of ovaries. But nonremoval of endometriomas might have certain drawbacks such as increase in the risk of infection, and rupture and follicular fluid contamination during oocyte retrieval. Both the European Society of Human Reproduction and Embryology (ESHRE) and RCOG have recommended surgical excision when an endometrioma has a diameter >3 cm as probably size more than this may cause difficulties during oocyte pick up. According to American Society for Reproductive Medicine (ASRM), there is doubt about any benefit of the excision procedure.[44] Surgery before IVF is also needed, if there is hydrosalpinx.

If salpingectomy is surgically challenging due to the extent of endometriotic disease, then proximal resection, clipping, or even aspiration at time of IVF can be the options.

For the women undergoing IVF, pretreatment includes surgery, expectant management, and medical treatment. According to a study, there is no significant effect on the rate of pregnancy and on the stimulation response of ovary when compared with no treatment.[35,45] However, some author observes that laparoscopic removal of endometriomas before IVF does not compromise the number or quality of oocytes obtained with COH, but at the same time, it does not improve fertility outcomes.[44] Hence, cystectomy may be an option when patient has pelvic pain as an associated symptom with infertility.

An ESHRE-sponsored survey[25] to learn the strategies employed for the management of endometrioma (>3 cm) prior to IVF found that surgical management was the most common treatment (82.2%), with cyst wall excision and drainage being the preferred surgical treatment (78.5%). The situation was different for women with previous ovarian surgery or recurrent endometrioma where surgical treatment was less commonly offered. Expectant management of endometrioma remains a major approach in these patients.

Women with normal ovarian reserve can be downregulated for prolonged period based on the study which shows that it may improve the rate of pregnancy compared to women with poor ovarian reserve.[46]

With regard to women who had previous ovarian surgery for endometrioma, implantation and clinical pregnancy rates were higher with the GnRH-agonist protocol than with the GnRH-antagonist protocol (22.6% and 39% vs. 15.9% and 27.5%, respectively). There was insufficient data to recommend surgical approach for the treatment of endometrioma in asymptomatic subfertile women. According to ESHRE guidelines, for <4 cm endometrioma and recurrence, expectant management is recommended. Women should be reassured that IVF does not influence the likelihood of endometriosis recurrence.[47,48]

> Recommendation—GCPR on Endometriosis-FOGSI:
> - In stages I and II, endometriosis patients undergoing laparoscopy before ART consider the complete surgical removal of endometriosis to improve live birth rate, although the benefit is not well-established (Evidence level C).[33]
> - In infertile women with endometrioma <3 cm, cystectomy prior to ART does not improve pregnancy rates (Evidence level A).[49]
> - In women with endometrioma >3 cm, cystectomy is indicated prior to ART when it is associated with pain or inaccessibility of follicles (Evidence level GPP).

## ASSISTED REPRODUCTION AND ENDOMETRIOSIS

### Intrauterine Insemination

There is evidence from several RCTs that controlled ovarian stimulation combined with intrauterine insemination (IUI) may be effective in improving fertility in patients with stages I and II endometriosis.

> Recommendation—GCPR on Endometriosis-FOGSI:
> - In stages I and II of endometriosis, treatment with super ovulation and IUI improves fertility compared to expectant management. Clinicians should take into consideration age, duration of infertility, ovarian reserve, and male factor (Evidence level A).[24]
> - Previous ovarian surgery results in longer stimulation, higher follicle-stimulating hormone (FSH) requirement, and decreased oocyte number, but no difference in fertilization and pregnancy outcome in subsequent ART cycles.

### In Vitro Fertilization

Assisted reproduction is widely used to manage infertility associated with endometriosis. IVF may enhance the low fecundity associated with advanced endometriosis. Various studies have reported beneficial effects,[15,16] while others have reported poor outcomes.[17-19] Various factors play a confounding role in pregnancy outcomes such as the size of endometrioma, previous medical treatment, surgical history, type of surgical treatment, time interval between procedure and embryo transfer, and skill of the surgeon. The mainstay of treatment for infertility due to endometriosis is IVF. Whether endometriomas need treatment before starting IVF is another topic of debate. When there is reduced response to gonadotropin hyperstimulation, it reflects damage to the ovarian reserve and is noted in patients with nonoperated endometrioma. At present, there is deficiency in randomized trials to consider the benefits of surgical treatment with respect to expectant management before IVF-ICSI (intracytoplasmic sperm injection) cycles. Patients with nonoperated unilateral endometrioma undergoing IVF can have a mean reduction of 25% (6–44%) in codominant follicles in the ovaries affected in comparison to the intact ones. Presence of large and multiple cysts in one ovary can further reduce responsiveness to exogenous gonadotropins.[20] Primordial follicles can be seen histologically close to the cyst wall, probably due to the technical difficulties encountered in removing the cyst, in >50% of the endometriomas removed.[50]

Pretreatment for 3–6 months with GnRH-a is suggested as it prevents the premature luteinizing hormone (LH) surge effect. The outcome of IVF-ET (embryo transfer) in patient with mild–moderate endometriosis after long protocol with GnRH-a and human menopausal gonadotropin (hMG) stimulation and tubal factor infertility is similar.[43]

Gonadotropin-releasing hormone antagonist could act as a reasonable choice for poor responder patients in IVF cycles as they cause immediate suppression of LH. Prolonged GnRH-a treatment prior to IVF in cases of moderate–severe endometriosishas been associated with increased pregnancy rates (recommendation grade A, evidence level E).[38]A Cochrane review analyzed three RCTs in women with endometriosis and compared those who received standard protocol versus GnRH agonist for 3–6 months.[51] However, this recommendation is based on only one properly randomized study and called for further research, particularly on the mechanism of action.

Management of severe/deeply infiltrating endometriosis is difficult and IVF with ultra-long or long protocol is mainstay when other treatments have failed. COH for IVF/ICSI is equally effective with both GnRH antagonist and GnRH agonist protocols in terms of implantation and clinical pregnancy rates, but COH with GnRH-a may be preferred because of the availability of more metaphase II (MII) oocyte and embryos. There is no evidence of increased cumulative endometriosis recurrence rates after ovarian stimulation for IVF/ICSI in women with endometriosis.

> **Recommendation—GCPR on Endometriosis-FOGSI:**
> - COS using GnRH agonists or antagonists is effective in IVF patients with mild-to-moderate endometriosis and in those with endometrioma who did not undergo surgery (Evidence level A).
> - IVF or ICSI is recommended when tubal function is impaired or in cases of advanced age or male infertility (Evidence level GPP).
> - IVF pregnancy rate and ovarian response to stimulation does not change significantly after surgical management of endometrioma (Evidence level A).[35,52]
> - In women undergoing IVF, stages III and IV are associated with poor implantation and lower clinical pregnancy rate (Evidence level A).[53]
> - In women with endometrioma, clinicians may use antibiotic prophylaxis at the time of oocyte retrieval to reduce the risk of ovarian abscess (Evidence level C).
> - In severe endometriosis, IVF treatment after surgery does not increase the risk of recurrence (Evidence level B).
> - The effectiveness of surgical removal of deeply infiltrating lesions in women undergoing ART with regards to pregnancy outcome is debatable (Evidence level C).

## Effect of Endometriosis on IVF Outcome

The IVF outcome in women with endometriosis varies with stages. The success rate of ART depends upon the severity of disease. A meta-analysis done by Harb et al. in 2013, including 27 observational studies with 8,984 women, compared the IVF outcomes in women with and without endometriosis undergoing IVF. The presence of severe endometriosis was associated with reduced implantation and clinical pregnancy rates, although the reduction in live birth rate was not statistically significant. The results in terms of implantation, clinical pregnancy, and live birth rates are higher in mild endometriosis.

The pregnancy rates are lower in endometriosis women compared to patients with tubal factor as per a meta-analysis by Barnhart et al.[54] The inferior IVF/ICSI outcomes of endometriosis women may be the result from decreased number of oocytes, poor quality of oocytes, development negative effect on embryogenesis, and implantation and impaired uterine receptivity, although IVF-ET remove critical steps in reproduction such as fertilization and early embryo development.

Ashrafi et al. observed a significantly poorer ovarian response to stimulation and lower number of MII oocytes retrieved among women with endometriomas as compared with a control group. Nevertheless, the quality of the embryos obtained and clinical pregnancy rates were comparable.

Reproductive outcomes among women undergoing IVF and diagnosed with endometriosis associated infertility do not differ significantly from women without the disease. Although women with endometriosis generate fewer oocytes, fertilization rate is not impaired, and the likelihood of achieving a live birth is also not affected.[54-56]

## CONCLUSION

In minimal–mild endometriosis, medical treatment of endometriosis does not improve spontaneous pregnancy rates, whereas there is evidence that surgery is beneficial. There is controversial evidence regarding endometrioma removal owing to the potential impact on ovarian reserve.

In moderate-to-severe endometriosis, whether surgical excision enhances pregnancy rate or not, RCTs or meta-analyses are needed. IUI is the treatment for minimal–mild endometriosis, doing ovarian stimulation is effective but the role of unstimulated IUI is uncertain.

In vitro fertilization treatment is advised in patients with male factor infertility and tubal factor. Pregnancy rates in tubal infertility are higher than endometriosis disease. Pretreatment for 3–6 months with GnRH agonist should be considered in endometriosis as it increases the rates of clinical pregnancy.

Combined medical, surgical, and ART treatments may benefit women and they should be used judiciously depending on the grade and the severity of endometriosis.

## FUTURE THOUGHTS

Endometriosis treatment is still in developing stage and various improvements in current medication such as oral GnRH antagonists and selective estrogen or progesterone receptor modulators need RCT. Especially in light of the fertility issues related to endometriosis, future therapies are being searched for that will manage pain symptoms without suppressing ovulation, or will result in cure rather than just temporary suppression of endometriosis. In this regard, immunomodulators and antiangiogenic agents are of prime interest. Obstacles to this research still involve lack of complete understanding of the pathogenesis and natural history of the disease.

## REFERENCES


1. Holoch KJ, Lessey BA. Endometrioisis and infertility. Clin Obstet Gynecol. 2010;53(2):429-38.
2. Schenken RS, Asch RH, Williams RF, Hodgen GD. Etiology of infertility in monkeys with endometriosis: luteinized unruptured follicles, luteal phase defects, pelvic adhesions and spontaneous abortions. Fertil Steril. 1984;41(1):122-30.
3. Kissler S, Hamscho N, Zangos S, Gatje R, Muller A, Rody A, et al. Diminished pregnancy rates in endometriosis due to impaired uterotubal transport assessed by hysterosalpingoscintigraphy. BJOG. 2005;112(10):1391-6.
4. Esmaeilzadeh S, Mirabi P, Basirat Z, Zeinalzadeh M, Khafri S. Association between endometriosis and hyperprolactinemia in infertile women. Iran J Reprod Med. 2015;13(3):155-60.
5. Wang H, Gorpudolo N, Behr B. The role of prolactin- and endometriosis-associated infertility. Obstet Gynecol Surv. 2009;64(8):542-7.
6. Mio Y, Toda T, Harada T, Terakawa N. Luteinized unruptured follicle in the early stages of endometriosis as a cause of unexplained infertility. Am J Obstet Gynecol. 1992;167(1):271-3.
7. Khorram O, Taylor RN, Ryan IP, Schall TJ, Landers DV. Peritoneal fluid concentrations of the cytokine RANTES correlate with the severity of endometriosis. Am J Obstet Gynecol.1993;169:1545-9.
8. Akoum A, Lemay A, McColl S, Turcot-Lemay L, Maheux R. Elevated concentration and biologic activity of monocyte chemotactic protein-1 in the peritoneal fluid of patients with endometriosis. Fertil Steril. 1996;66(1):17-23.
9. Arici A, Oral E, Attar E, Tazuke SI, Olive DL. Monocyte chemotactic protein-1 concentration in peritoneal fluid of women with endometriosis and its modulation of expression in mesothelial cells. Fertil Steril. 1997;67(6):1065-72.
10. Hornung D, Dohrn K, Sotlar K, Greb RR, Wallwiener D, Keisel L, et al. Localization in tissues and secretion of eotaxin by cells from normal endometrium and endometriosis. J Clin Endocrinol Metab. 2000;85(7):2604-8.
11. Ryan IP, Tseng JF, Schriock ED, Khorram O, Landers DV, Taylor RN. Interleukin-8 concentrations are elevated in peritoneal fluid of women with endometriosis. Fertil Steril. 1995;63(4):929-32.
12. Mueller MD, Mazzucchelli L, Buri C, Lebovic DI, Dreher E, Taylor RN. Epithelial neutrophil-activating peptide 78 concentrations are elevated in the peritoneal fluid of women with endometriosis. Fertil Steril. 2003;79(Suppl 1):815-20.
13. Lessey BA, Castelbaum AJ, Sawin SW, Buck CA, Schinnar R, Bilker W, et al. Aberrant integrin expression in the endometrium of women with endometriosis. J Clin Endocrinol Metab. 1994;79(2):643-9.

14. Cho S, Park SH, Choi YS, Seo SK, Kim HY, Park KH, et al. Expression of cyclooxygenase-2 in eutopic endometrium and ovarian endometriotic tissue in women with severe endometriosis. Gynecol Obstet Invest. 2010;69(2):93-100.

15. Lebovic DI, Mueller MD, Taylor RN. Immunobiology of endometriosis. Fertil Steril. 2001;75(1):1-10.

16. Karita M, Yamashita Y, Hayashi A, Yoshida Y, Hayashi M, Yamamoto H, et al. Does advanced-stage endometriosis affects the gene expression of estrogen and progesterone receptors in granulosa cells? Fertil Steril. 2011;95(3):889-94.

17. Talwar P. Endometriosis andinfertility. Indian Fertil Soc. 2017;2(2):15.

18. Adamson GD, Pasta DJ. Endometriosis fertility index: the new, validated endometriosis staging system. Fertil Steril. 2010;94(5);1609-15.

19. Hughes E, Brown J, Collins JJ, Farquhar C, Fedorkow DM, Vandekerckhove P. Ovulation suppression for endometriosis for women with subfertility. Cochrane Database Syst Rev. 2007:CD000155.

20. Alborzi S, Ravanbakhsh R, Parsanezhad E, Alborzi M, Alborzi S, Dehbashi S. A comparison of follicular response of ovaries to ovulation induction after laparoscopic ovarian cystectomy or fenestration and coagulation versus normal ovaries in patient with ovarian endometrioma. Fertil Steril. 2007;88(2):507-9.

21. Patel BG, Rudnicki M, Yu J, Shu Y, Taylor RN. Progesterone resistance in endometriosis: origins, consequences and interventions. Acta Obstet Gynecol Scand. 2017;96(6):623-32.

22. Schindler AE. Dienogest in long-term treatment of endometriosis. Int J Womens Health. 2011;3:175-84.

23. National Collaborating Centre for Women's and Children's Health (UK). Fertility: Assessment and Treatment for People with Fertility Problems. London (UK): RCOG Press; 2004, 2017.

24. Verma S. Evidence linked treatment for endometriosis associated infertility. Apollo Med. 2012;9(3):184-92.

25. Yap C, Furness S, Farquhar C. Pre- and postoperative medical therapy for endometriosis surgery. Cochrane Database Syst Rev. 2004;(3):CD003678.

26. Kriplani A, Devi R. Good Clinical Practice Recommendations on Endometriosis-FOGSI; 2016.

27. Winkel CA. Evaluation and management of women with endometriosis. Obstet Gynecol. 2003;102(2):397-408.

28. Marcoux S, Maheux R, Berube S. Laparoscopic surgery in infertile women with minimal or mild endometriosis. Canadian Collaborative Group on Endometriosis. N Engl J Med. 1997;337(4):217-22.

29. Royal College of Obstetricians and Gynaecologists. The investigation and management of endometriosis (green-top guideline; no. 24). London: RCOG; 2006:3.

30. Exacoustos C, Zupi E, Amadio A, Szabolcs B, De Vivo B, Marconi D, et al. Laparoscopic removal of endometriomas: sonographic evaluation of residual functioning ovarian tissue. Am J Obstet Gynecol. 2004;191(1):68-72.

31. Yun BH, Choi YS, Lee BS. Management of endometriosis-associated infertility. J Androl Gynaecol. 2014;2(2):7.

32. Jacobson TZ, Duffy JM, Barlow D, Farquhar C, Koninckx PR, Olive D. Laparoscopic surgery for subfertility associated with endometriosis. Cochrane Database Syst Rev. 2010;(1):CD001398.

33. Opøien HK, Fedorcsak P, Byholm T, Tanbo T. Complete surgical removal of minimal and mild endometriosis improves outcome of subsequent IVF/ICSI treatment. Reprod Biomed Online. 2011;23(3):389-95.

34. Dunselman GA, Vermeulen N, Becker C, Calhaz-Jorge C, D'Hooghe T, De Bie B, et al. ESHRE guideline: management of women with endometriosis. Hum Reprod Oxf Engl. 2014;29(3):400-12.

35. Tsoumpou I, Kyrgiou M, Gelbaya TA, Nardo LG. The effect of surgical treatment for endometrioma on in vitro fertilization outcomes: a systematic review and meta-analysis. Fertil Steril. 2009;92(1):75-87.

36. Hornstein MD, Yuzpe AA, Burry KA, Heinrichs LR, Buttram VL Jr, Orwoll ES. Prospective randomised double-blind trial of 3 versus 6 months of nafarelin therapy for endometriosis associated pelvic pain. Fertil Steril. 1995;63(5):955-62.

37. Kampe D, Sahl AC, Schweppe K-W. Pra- und postoperative Endometriose therapiemit GnRH-Agonisten in Depotform: drei- versus sechsmonatige Behandlungsdauer. Zentralbl Gynakol. 2003;125:304.

38. Bansal K. Manual of Endometriosis. New Delhi: Jaypee Brothers Medical Publishers; 2013. pp. 193-7.

39. Al-Azemi M, Bernal AL, Steele J, Gramsbergen I, Barlow D, Kennedy S. Ovarian response to repeated controlled stimulation in in-vitro fertilization cycles in patients with ovarian endometriosis. Human Reprod. 2000;15(1):72-5.

40. Hart R, Hickey M, Maouris P, Buckett W, Garry R. Excisional surgery versus ablative surgery for ovarian endometriomata: a Cochrane Review. Hum Reprod. 2005;20(11):3000-7.

41. Alborzi S, Momtahan M, Parsanezhad ME, Dehbashi S, Zolghadri J, Alborzi S. A prospective, randomized study comparing laparoscopic ovarian cystectomy versus fenestration and coagulation in patients with endometriomas. Fertil Steril. 2004;82(6):1633-7.

42. Garcia-Velasco JA, Mahutte NG, Corona J, Zuniga V, Giles J, Arici A, et al. Removal of endometriomas before in vitro fertilization does not improve fertility outcomes: a matched, case–control study. Fertil Steril. 2004;81(5):1194-7.

43. Somigliana E, Ragni G, Benedetti F, Borroni R, Vegetti W, Crosignani PG. Does laparoscopic excision of endometriotic ovarian cysts significantly affect ovarian reserve? Insights from IVF cycles. Hum Reprod. 2003;18(11):2450-3.

44. Suganuma N, Wakahara Y, Ishida D, Asano M, Kitagawa T, Katsumata Y, et al. Pretreatment for ovarian endometrial cyst before in vitro fertilization. Gynecol Obstet Invest. 2002;54(Suppl 1):36-40; discussion 41-2.

45. Demirol A, Guven S, Baykal C, Gurgan T. Effect of endometrioma cystectomy on IVF outcome: a prospective randomized study. Reprod Biomed Online. 2006;12(5):639-43.

46. Klinkert ER, Broekmans FJM, Looman CWN, Habbema JDF, te Velde ER. Expected poor responders on the basis of an antral follicle count do not benefit from a higher starting dose of gonadotrophins in IVF treatment: a randomized controlled trial. Hum Reprod. 2005;20(3):611-5.

47. Canis M, Pouly JL, Tamburro S, Mage G, Wattiez A, Bruhat MA. Ovarian response during IVF-embryo transfer cycles after laparoscopic ovarian cystectomy for endometriotic cysts of >3 cm in diameter. Hum Reprod. 2001;16(12):2583-6.

48. Marconi G, Vilela M, Quintana R, Sueldo C. Laparoscopic ovarian cystectomy of endometriomas does not affect the ovarian response to gonadotropin stimulation. Fertil Steril. 2002;78(4):876-8.

49. Benschop L, Farquhar C, van der Poel N, Heineman MJ. Interventions for women with endometrioma prior to assisted reproductive technology. In: Cochrane Database of Systematic Reviews. John Wiley & Sons, Ltd; 2010.

50. Hachisuga T, Kawarabayashi T. Histopathological analysis of laparoscopically treated ovarian endometriotic cysts with special reference to loss of follicles. Hum Reprod. 2002;17(2):432-5.

51. Ho HY, Lee RK, Hwu YM, Lin MH, Su JT, Tsai YC. Poor response of ovaries with endometrioma previously treated with cystectomy to control ovarian hyperstimulation. J Assst Reprod Genet. 2002;19(11):507-11.

52. Dong X, Wang R, Zheng Y, Xiong T, Liao X, Huang B, et al. Surgical treatment for endometrioma does not increase clinical pregnancy rate or live birth/ongoing pregnancy rate after fresh IVF/ICSI treatment. Am J Transl Res. 2014;6(2):163-8.

53. Kuivasaari P, Hippeläinen M, Anttila M, Heinonen S. Effect of endometriosis on IVF/ICSI outcome: stage III/IV endometriosis worsens cumulative pregnancy and live-born rates. Hum Reprod. 2005;20(11):3130-5.

54. Barnhart K, Dunsmoor-Su R, Coutifaris C. Effect of endometriosis on in vitro fertilization. Fertil Steril. 2002;77(6):1148-55.

55. Harb HM, Gallos ID, Chu J, Harb M, Coomarasamy A. The effect of endometriosis on in vitro fertilisation outcome: a systematic review and meta-analysis. BJOG. 2013;120(11):1308-20.

56. Ashrafi M, Fakheri T, Kiani K, Sadeghi M, Akhoond MR. Impact of the endometrioma on ovarian response and pregnancy rate in in vitro fertilization cycles. Int J Fertil Steril. 2014;8(1):29-34.

# CHAPTER 9

# Endometrioma

Neharika Malhotra Bora, Astha Ubeja, Narendra Malhotra, Jaideep Malhotra

## INTRODUCTION

Endometriosis is a chronic gynecologic disease characterized by endometrial-like tissue outside the uterus.[1] When this tissue grows to form a cyst inside the ovaries is termed as endometrioma **(Fig. 1)**. This may cause chronic pelvic pain during periods and also have an effect on reproduction.[2] Despite its recognition for centuries, it is still a mystery to completely understand its pathogenesis **(Fig. 2)**. But investigations employing modern molecular methods are yielding new insights of the disease. It is found in 20% of asymptomatic women, 30% with infertility and in up to 50% with pain symptoms.[3]

In the women at reproductive age, the prevalence of ovarian endometrioma is frequent. In the treatment for endometrioma, the effect of medical management is not suggested and not applicable. According to recommendation, if the size of endometrioma is more than 4 cm, has to be removed. This will help in pain reduction and can also increase spontaneous conception rates. Cystectomy can be choice of treatment but it can lead to damage to ovaries and even recurrence risk if ablation is incompletely done.

The immunobiology of endometriosis has been shown in **Figure 3**.

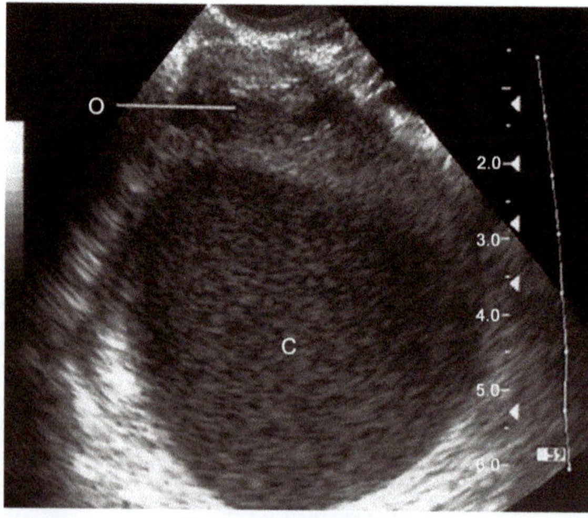

**Fig. 1:** Endometrioma.

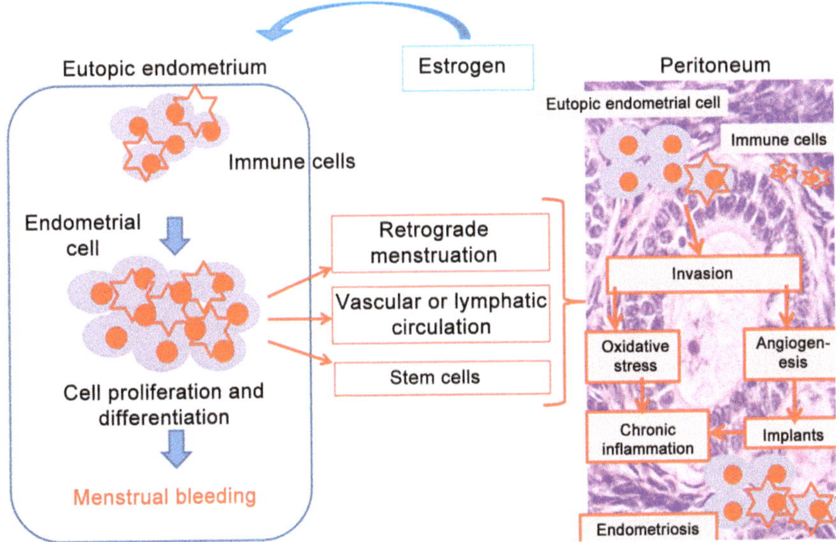


**Fig. 2:** Pathogenesis.

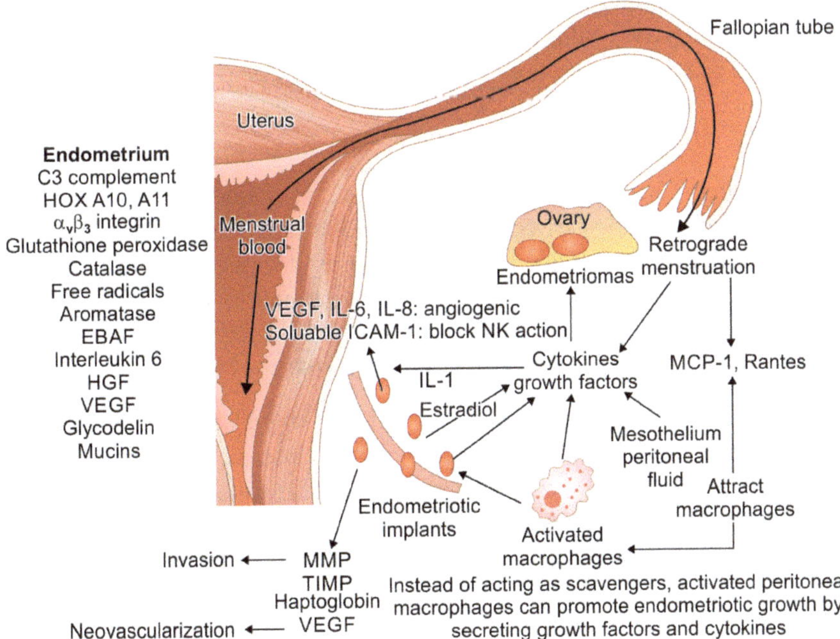


**Fig. 3:** Immunobiology of endometriosis.

## DIAGNOSIS

The clinical symptoms include dysmenorrhea, nonmenstrual pelvic pain, dyspareunia, dyschezia, cyclic bowel and bladder symptoms, infertility, and

| **Table 1:** Symptoms of endometriosis and rate of occurrence. | |
|---|---|
| Dysmenorrhea | 60–80% |
| Chronic pelvic pain | 40–50% |
| Deep dyspareunia | 40–50% |
| Infertility | 30–50% |
| Severe menstrual pain and irregular flow and/or premenstrual spotting | 10–20% |
| Tenesmus, dyschezia, hematochezia, costiveness, or diarrhea | 1–2% |
| Dysuria, pollakiuria, micro- or macroscopic hematuria | 1–2% |
| *Source:* Bulletti C, Coccia ME, Battistoni S, Borini A. Endometriosis and infertility. J Assist Reprod Genet. 2010;27(8):441-7. | |

chronic fatigue. It differs a lot and hence; none of the presenting signs or symptoms are pathognomonic for this disease **(Table 1)**.

## Pelvic Pain

In women, the prevention of pelvic pain is a general. In endometriosis, the main symptom is pain but to diagnose the actual reason is difficult. Because the cause and source of pain varies, it cannot be used as endometriosis marker. Types of pain include dysmenorrhea, chronic pelvic pain, chronic nonmenstrual pelvic pain, and dyspareunia.[4] Dysmenorrhea and pain that are new in onset, progressive or severe strongly suggest endometriosis.

## Infertility

Endometriosis can lead to infertility in women at reproductive age. According to a case-control study carried out in the United Kingdom; it was found that the infertility is 6 times more in women diagnosed with endometriosis.[5] The causes of infertility in endometriosis have been shown in **Table 2**.

## Other Symptomatic Indicators of Endometriosis

There are studies showing other risk factors linked with endometriosis, which exhibit related factors like increased blood loss, increased cycle length and duration of bleeding, cycles may be shorter, irregular menstrual cycles, postcoital bleeding, and dyschezia.[5] These findings may not be consistent, a collection of such related symptoms may indicate endometriosis.

## Physical Examination

Diagnosis of endometriosis by a physical examination is not effective as compare to surgical diagnosis as per many studies.[6] Physical findings vary widely in endometriosis. In ovarian endometriomas, patient can have a fixed tender adnexal mass. Focal tenderness, thickening and nodularity of the uterosacral ligaments are also a common finding.

**Table 2:** Causes of infertility in endometriosis.

| Ovulatory dysfunction | Interference with implantation |
|---|---|
| Abnormal folliculogenesis<br>An ovulation<br>Luteal phase defect<br>Luteinized unruptured follicle syndrome | Endometrial dysfunction |
| *Immunological alterations* | *Mechanical factors* |
| Decreased sperm survival<br>Altered immunity | Anatomical distortion of tubes<br>Altered tubal motility<br>Interference with ovum pick up<br>Peritubal adhesions |
| *Peritoneal factors* | *Interference with coital function* |
| Intraperitoneal inflammation<br>Local production of prostaglandins/Cytokines | Dyspareunia |
|  | *Sperm inactivation* |
|  | Phagocytosis by macrophages<br>Inactivation by antibodies |

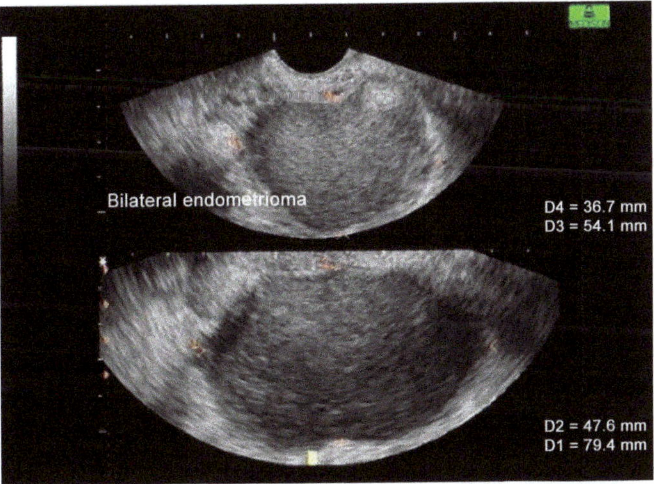


**Fig. 4:** Ultrasound image showing endometrioma.

## IMAGING STUDIES IN CLINICAL DIAGNOSIS

### Ultrasonography

Ultrasonography (USG) is an imaging technique which uses high-frequency ultrasound waves. USG helps to diagnose endometriosis and adenomyosis which causes pain and infertility. The severity of disease can be found by transvaginal sonography (TVS). Difference between endometrioma and simple cyst can be reveal by the morphology seen in USG **(Fig. 4)**.

On USG, ovarian endometrioma is a round, *homogeneous, hypoechoic cyst with or without internal septa and with poor vascularization of the cyst wall.*[1] The differential diagnosis of other adnexal mass includes luteal cysts, cystadenomas, pyosalpinges, dermoids, and ovarian cancers, because, in these masses, the cyst content (blood, mucus or pus) may display low-level echoes on ultrasound.[7]

Luteal and ovarian cancers cysts are rich vascularization of the wall and there is arterial flow within papillary projections and echogenic areas of the cyst while endometriotic cysts are related with scanty vascularization of the cyst wall.[8] Ovaries with bilateral endometrioma are called kissing ovaries as they are found adhering to each other behind or above the uterus. For evaluation of endometriosis, transvaginal ultrasound (TVUS) is considered the first-line imaging.

## Magnetic Resonance Imaging

Magnetic resonance imaging (MRI) is advised when USG findings are equivocal and in specific patients. MRI is an expensive procedure and hence not used frequently. MRI is helpful in ureteral involvement and to detect extensive adhesions in the pelvis **(Fig. 5)**.[9]

## OTHER MARKERS

Patients with endometriosis were found to have lower *anti-Müllerian hormone* (AMH) serum levels. There is a correlation between the severity of the disease and AMH levels. This can be useful in controlled ovarian stimulation in women with severe endometriosis. Cancer antigen 125 (CA 125) assay is used to confirm endometriosis. Human epididymis protein (HE4) assay could differentiate between ovarian endometriosis cysts from

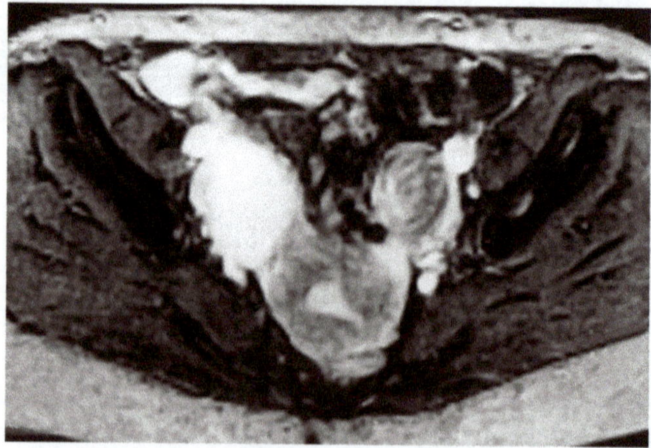

**Fig. 5:** Magnetic resonance imaging (MRI) showing endometrioma.

malignant. Molecular tests are also available to analyze at genetic level and identify the gene responsible for endometriosis.

## SURGICAL DIAGNOSIS

Laparoscopy with histological examination of excised lesion has traditionally been the gold standard for the diagnosis of endometriosis. Endometriomas appear as smooth dark cyst associated with adhesions and containing a dense brown chocolate-like fluid. Larger endometriomas are usually multilocular. They are accompanied by dense adhesions and deep infiltrating endometriosis.[10]

## MANAGEMENT

### Surgical Management of Endometriosis

1. Laparoscopy:
    a. Conservative treatment:
        - Laparoscopic aspiration
        - Cystectomy:
            - Intraperitoneal cystectomy (IPC)
            - Transperitoneal cystectomy (TPC)
            - Laser or bipolar coagulation of the inner lining
            - Three-stage management
    b. Radical treatment:
        - Ovariectomy
        - Adnexectomy.
2. Laparotomy.

### Aspiration: Ultrasound Guided

In this procedure, under the guidance of vaginal USG, needle is inserted in the endometrioma and aspiration is done. It is a feasible procedure but may lead to adhesions, complications, injury to ovary and recurrence.[11]

*Cystectomy, surgery under laparoscopy* guidance, will allow diagnosis, staging, and treatment. Cystectomy or fenestration and coagulation, radical treatment—ovariectomy or adnexectomy are used for treatment of endometrioma.

Removal of endometrioma > 4 cm is significant in pain reduction and to increase the rate of spontaneous conception. There is no evidence showing effect on in vitro fertilization (IVF) success with presence of small endometriomas. The objective is to remove all the implants and endometrioma without damaging the ovaries.[10] Superficial endometriosis lesions present as adhesions, and restore the involved organs to a normal anatomic and physiologic condition. Endometriomas must be treated by laparoscopy **(Figs. 6A and B)**.

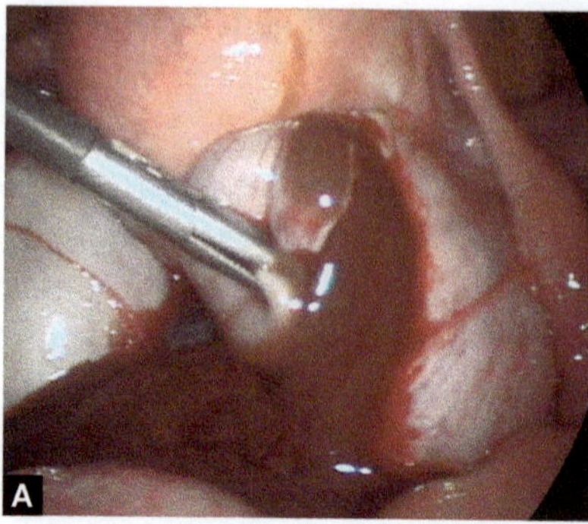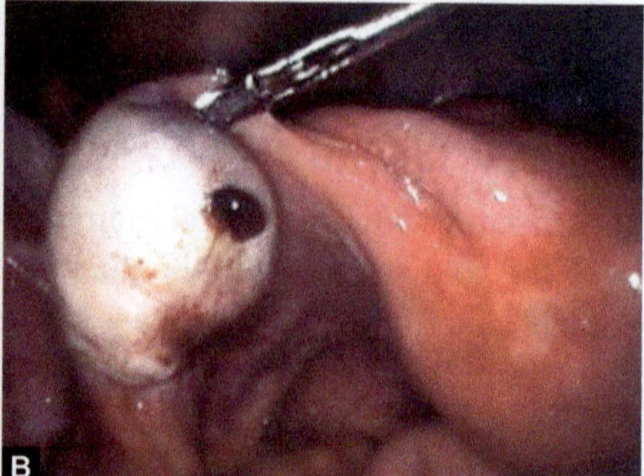

**Figs. 6A and B:** Laparoscopic excision.

As conservative treatment, cystectomy is considered as first line. For eradication of endometriosis, surgical resection of endometriomas, by laparoscopy or laparotomy, is effective but with high risk of recurrence.

## Fulguration

When the size of endometrioma is 2 cm or less, coagulation of the implants with laser-ablated, or is excised with the help of scissors, biopsy forceps, or electrodes. For the best treatment, all lesions which are visible at ovarian surface have to be removed. Due to the heterogeneous appearance, it is difficult for clinicians to diagnose endometriotic implants.[12] For confirmation of disease, the diagnosis has to be definite and confirm by the presence of at least two of the following: (1) endometrial glands, (2) endometrial stroma, and (3) hemosiderin-laden macrophages.

## CONCLUSION

Management of ovarian endometrioma is inefficient by medications and hence cannot be advised. Laparoscopy is the gold standard for diagnosis as well as the management with respect to endometriomas. Preoperative medical treatment is also not suggested for endometrioma. For infertility also postoperative medications have no benefits. Assisted reproductive technology (ART) is indicated for the treatment of infertility after surgery. Recurrence and pain also does not have any effect of medications. Individualized treatment has to be advised in endometriosis.

## REFERENCES


1. Savelli L. Transvaginal sonography for the assessment of ovarian and pelvic endometriosis: how deep is our understanding? Ultrasound Obstet Gynecol. 2009;33:497-501.
2. Chapron C, Vercellini P, Barakat H, Vieira M, Dubuisson JB. Management of ovarian endometriomas. Hum Reprod Update. 2002;8(6):591-7.

3. Leyland N, Casper R, Laberge P, Singh SS, SOGC. Endometriosis: diagnosis and management. J Obstet Gynaecol Can. 2010;32:S1-32.

4. Schliep KC, Mumford SL, Peterson CM, Chen Z, Johnstone EB, Sharp HT, et al. Pain typology and incident endometriosis. Hum Reprod. 2015;30:2427-38.

5. Ashrafi M, Sadatmahalleh SJ, Akhoond MR, Talebi M. Evaluation of risk factors associated with endometriosis in infertile women. Int J Fertil Steril. 2016;10:11-21.

6. Eskenazi B, Warner M, Bonsignore L, Olive D, Samuels S, Vercellini P. Validation study of nonsurgical diagnosis of endometriosis. Fertil Steril. 2001;76:929-35.

7. Valentin L. Use of morphology to characterize and manage common adnexal masses. Best Pract Res Clin Obstet Gynaecol. 2004;18:71-89.

8. Guerriero S, Ajossa S, Mais V, Risalvato A, Lai MP, Melis GB. The diagnosis of endometriomas using color Doppler energy imaging. Hum Reprod. 1998;13:1691-5.

9. Bianek-Bodzak A, Szurowska E, Sawicki S, Liro M. The importance and perspective of magnetic resonance imaging in the evaluation of endometriosis. Biomed Res Int. 2013;2013:436589.

10. Fernando S, Soh PQ, Cooper M, Evans S, Reid G, Tsaltas J, et al. Reliability of visual diagnosis of endometriosis. J Minim Invasive Gynecol. 2013;20:783-9.

11. Zanetta G, Lissoni A, Dalla Valle C, Trio D, Pittelli M, Rangoni G. Ultrasound-guided aspiration of endometriomas: possible applications and limitations. Fertil Steril. 1995;64:709-13.

12. Buchweitz O, Poel T, Diedrich K, Malik E. The diagnostic dilemma of minimal and mild endometriosis under routine conditions. J Am Assoc Gynecol Laparosc. 2003;10:85-9.

# CHAPTER 10

# Rectosigmoid Endometriosis/Deep Infiltrating Endometriosis

*Kuldeep Jain, Maansi Jain*

## INTRODUCTION

Endometriosis is an enigmatic disease because neither the etiology nor the natural history, nor the precise mechanisms of the associated pelvic pain and/or infertility are completely understood. Endometriosis can be divided into three broad categories:[1]

1. Peritoneal or surface endometriosis
2. Endometrioma
3. Deep infiltrating endometriosis (DIE).

Each of these varieties may occur alone or coexist with other forms.[2] DIE is a specific entity, unique in terms of origin, location, histology, and clinical symptoms. DIE is the presence of one or more endometriotic nodules deeper than 5 mm. In a study at a large tertiary care center, 40% of patients with endometriosis had deep disease. DIE is associated with more severe pain and infertility. In patients with endometriosis, diagnosis is commonly made 7–9 years after the initial pelvic pain presentation. For these reasons, well-directed history taking and proper evaluation and treatment should be pursued to relieve pain and optimize outcomes. Deep lesions are considered very active and are strongly associated with pelvic pain symptoms. [The definition of deep endometriosis includes rectovaginal lesions as well as infiltrative forms that involve vital structures like bowel, ureters, and bladder.] Deeply infiltrating endometriosis should probably be considered as a specific type of endometriosis different from superficial (and active) and intermediate (and inactive) endometriosis and from endometriomas. First, deep endometriosis is strongly associated with pelvic pain, almost all women with lesions deeper than 1 cm suffering badly. Second, the secretion of CA-125 by superficial endometriosis is directed mainly toward the peritoneal fluid, whereas deep endometriosis secretes more toward the bloodstream. Third, deep endometriosis is morphologically a very active disease, whereas at intermediate depths, endometriosis is more inactive. Fourth, the biphasic frequency distribution pattern suggests that deep endometriosis is another entity.

The prevalence of endometriosis and the DIE seems to have increased over past two decades. This may be due to a growing awareness and also a quicker referral. Studies report that 15–30% women with endometriosis will have deep infiltrating disease as well, although this might vary according to the referral patterns.[3,4] Mostly, a deep endometriosis is associated with other forms of the disease like superficial implants, endometriotic ovarian cysts, and/or pelvic adhesions. In one study, an isolated deep endometriosis in absence of other endometriotic lesions was present in only 6.5%.[5] Urinary tract endometriosis is a rare entity, affecting approximately 1–2% of all cases of endometriosis,[6] while ureteral involvement is seen in 0.1–0.4% of all cases of endometriosis.[7]

## PATHOGENESIS

The mechanism by which endometriosis develops is still subject of research:

- *Sampson's theory of retrograde menstruation*: This is the most popular theory. This theory explains retrograde flow of menstrual blood from uterus through fallopian tubes into the peritoneal cavity. Endometrial fragments get implanted onto peritoneal surface at dependent sites like ovaries, uterosacral ligaments, and pouch of Douglas (POD). Although this theory can explain pelvic endometriosis, it fails to explain distant endometriosis.

- *Halban's theory of lymphatic spread*: This theory can explain endometriosis inflicting pelvic lymph nodes. This theory proposes that endometrial tissue can metastasize through the draining lymph channels of uterus to the lymph nodes.

- *Meyer and Ivanoff theory of coelomic metaplasia*: Mesothelial cells from peritoneal and ovarian surfaces may undergo metaplasia to endometrial tissue. This can occur due to chronic irritation by the menstrual blood. Stem cells can also transform into endometrial tissue under hyperestrogenic state.

- *Direct implantation theory*: This theory postulates that endometrial cells can directly get implanted at new sites and grow like abdominal scar after hysterotomy, cesarean section or myomectomy, and episiotomy scars.

- *Vascular theory*: This is the least explained theory, but it can explain endometriosis at distant sites like lungs and brain.

- *Genetic theory*: Genes responsible for increased susceptibility have been found to be *EMX2*—a transcriptional factor encoding proteins for reproductive tract development and *PTEN*—a tumor suppressor gene responsible for malignant transformation to endometrioid adenocarcinoma in ovarian endometriosis. Both these genes are located within or near *20p13* locus. Other genes implicated are those encoding for interleukin-15, glycodelin, Dickkopf-1, semaphoring E, aromatase, progesterone receptor, and multiple angiogenic factors.

- *Biomolecular theory*: Endometriosis patients have an impaired immune system response, increased production of cytokines and proinflammatory mediators, increased over all angiogenic activity, excessive estrogen production, and progesterone resistance.
- *Environment theory*: The most important toxins are dioxins (e.g., *TCDD— 2,3,7,8-tetrachlorodibenzo-p-dioxin*). These are byproducts of industrial processing and often enter our body through food chain. These promote somatic mutation of endometrium by acting as transcription factors promoting increased interleukins synthesis, activation of *cytochrome P450*, and alteration of tissue remodeling.

## HISTOPATHOLOGY

Infiltration by endometrial glands and stroma occurs into adjacent fibromuscular tissue along the loose connective tissue and that penetration is arrested at the border of the underlying fat tissue. Hyperplasia of the surrounding smooth muscle and fibrous tissue results in nodule formation and, important, DIE is focally associated with microendometriomas of 500–2,000 μm in diameter particularly in the submucosal layer of the vagina, rectum, or bladder. These non-OMAs (ovarian microendometrioma) are also lined, similarly to the OMA, by endometrial surface epithelium with or without stroma or by polypoid endometriotic tissue.[8]

Fibrosis appears as the phenomenon underpinning endometriosis-associated morbidity and some manifestations of the disease (i.e., adhesions). Fibrosis seems to represent a self-amplifying event of endometriosis.

Deep infiltrating endometriosis is predominantly composed of fibrotic tissue. DIE should be called deep fibrotic endometriosis. Deep endometriotic nodules were histologically composed of scanty stroma and glandular epithelium disseminated in extensive fibromuscular tissue.[9] Myofibroblasts are contractile nonmuscle cells that are usually activated in response to injury with the intent to repair damaged extracellular matrix (ECM). A persistent myofibroblast activity causes accumulation and contraction of collagenous ECM, a condition called fibrosis. Macroscopically, due to accumulation of ECM, contraction of myofibroblasts, and reduced vasculature, fibrotic organs, usually display an uneven surface, are pale and not elastic. This process ultimately results in disruption of the normal anatomical structure.[10]

**What are the various locations?**
The DIE implants are located in various specific locations as given below:
- In the posterior cul-de-sac area[11]
- The intestinal system
- The urinary system
- Uterosacral ligaments[12]

- Retrocervical area of uterus where uterosacral ligaments join together, known as carina of uterus[13]
- The posterior vaginal wall
- The anterior rectal wall.[14]

The most common sites for DIE are the rectovaginal space and the rectosigmoid area; most of women suffer infiltration of endometriotic lesions in these areas.[15] Out of all cases of DIE, the uterosacral ligaments involvement is seen in 69.2% cases, vagina is involved in 14.5% cases, intestinal system is involved in 9.9% cases, and bladder is involved in approximately 6.4% cases.[11]

## CLASSIFICATION OF DEEP INFILTRATING ENDOMETRIOSIS

The importance of location of the deeply infiltrating endometriotic lesions cannot be overemphasized, as the success of the any surgical operation depends on how radical the surgical removal is done.[16] A classification based on the anatomic location of endometriotic lesions had been suggested by Chapron C et al.[11]

- *A: Anterior DIE—*
  - A1: Bladder
- *P: Posterior DIE—*
  - P1: Uterosacral ligament
  - P2: Vagina
  - P3: Intestine.

*Subclassification of retroperitoneal lesions by locations (precisely defined with transrectal USG and MRI):*

- *Type I: Rectovaginal septum lesions (10%)—*
  - They are usually small and situated within the rectovaginal septum between the posterior wall of the vaginal mucosa and the anterior wall of the rectal muscularis. The lesion is situated under the peritoneal fold of the cul-de-sac of Douglas.[17]
- *Type II: Posterior wall fornix lesions (65%)—*
  - The posterior fornix is retrocervical and corresponds to the vaginal wall and to the posterior wall of the posterior lip of the cervix. These lesions are often small, and there is no extension to the rectovaginal septum or rectal wall.[17]
- *Type III: Hourglass-shaped lesions (25%)—*
  - Hourglass-shaped lesions are usually larger lesions > 3 cm, with a greater risk of extension to the rectal wall; there is cranial extension of posterior forniceal lesions on to the anterior rectal wall giving it the shape of hourglass. Infiltration of the rectal muscularis is usually the rule in this variety and the lesion is always situated beneath the fold of rectovaginal pouch.[17]

Another classification is based on the primary organ involvement. Major types of DIE based on organ involvement are:

- *Intestinal DIE*: Infiltration of endometriotic lesion into the bowel, at least up to muscular layer, is termed as intestinal DIE. Rectosigmoid colon is the most common affected part.[11] The initial lesion starts in the dependent part of POD where inflammation leads to formation of adhesions and invasion into muscular layer of bowel anteriorly and into the vagina. Further infiltration into uterosacral ligament and adhesion formation leads to partial or complete obliteration of POD. Clinical presentation is intense pelvic pain, pain and bleeding during defecation, and deep dyspareunia leading to loss of libido. In severe case, patient may complain of cyclical rectal bleeding. Further invasion may lead to stenosis, signs of partial obstruction though very rare.

- *Bladder endometriosis*: Endometriosis of bladder is defined as infiltration of muscular layer of the urinary bladder.[11] The anterior cul-de-sac may become obliterated due to extensive adhesions between anterior wall of uterus and uterovesical peritoneal fold. Patients with deep infiltration often present with dysuria and cyclical hematuria depending on the depth of invasion. A detrusor nodule may be palpated usually during surgery, near the dome, and above the isthmus.

- *Ureteric endometriosis*: Incidence of ureteric involvement is quite low (0.1–0.4%) of all cases of endometriosis. Endometriosis of the ureter is of two types—extrinsic and intrinsic type.[18] Extrinsic type is more common, usually associated with bilateral endometrioma, compressing the ureter by encircling the surroundings and causing obstruction; while intrinsic type is rare and involves all layers of ureter.[19] Presentation in these cases ranges from nonspecific pain, renal obstruction, unilateral or bilateral hydronephrosis, and loss of renal function in affected kidney.

## CLINICAL PRESENTATION

Various presenting symptoms are related to affected organ, but all patients have severe chronic pelvic pain. Apart from pain, painful defecation, renal/urinary symptoms, and infertility, prevalence of different clinical features as reported by two large studies are discussed in **Table 1**.

Only 3.7% patients had cyclical bleeding and/or pain on defecation during the menstrual period.

Presenting symptoms are most often related to location of disease, but the relationship is not absolute in nature:

- Deep dyspareunia and constant perineal pain—uterosacral ligament
- Painful defecation, noncyclic pelvic pain, menstrual blood on stools, menstrual diarrhea, intestinal DIE, and posterior DIE

**Table 1:** Prevalence of different clinical features as reported by two large studies.

|  | *Bellelis et al. 892 cases of DIE* | *Gernot et al. 200 cases of DIE[20]* |
|---|---|---|
| • Chronic pelvic pain | 56.8% | 22% |
| • Deep dyspareunia | 54.7% | 34.5% |
| • Cyclical intestinal complaints | 48.3% | 14.5% |
| • Incapacitating dysmenorrhea | 28.4% | 77.5% |
| • Cyclical urinary complaints | 11.7% | 2% |

- Dysuria, lower urinary tract symptoms, recurrent cystitis in premenstrual period, hematuria—bladder endometriosis
- Severe dysmenorrhea—adhesions in the Douglas of pouch and rectal or vaginal infiltration.

Apart from these symptoms, DIE patients are more prone to be depressive, mood alteration, or anxiety disorders, which can be seen in as high as 60% cases. Thus, a detailed history should be taken in these cases to quantify the severity and location of disease.

## DIAGNOSIS

### Clinical Examination

A rectovaginal bimanual examination is useful to diagnose the deep-seated nodule or thickness in rectovaginal septum; however, the accuracy of clinical diagnosis of DIE is very limited. Rectal examination is important in suspected cases of rectal endometriosis. Presence of thickening of fornices or posterior pouch and presence of nodule or deep tenderness are all pathognomonic of DIE.

### Imaging Techniques

Imaging techniques like transvaginal sonography (TVS), transrectal ultrasonography (TRUS), and MRI are available but all have limitations. TVS remains the primary modality of imaging but the sensitivity for DIE is low in the absence of endometrioma as per endometriosis special interest group of European Society of Human Reproduction and Embryology (ESHRE).[21] TVS also has a role in diagnosing bladder or rectum endometriosis. The USG has limitations in diagnosing peritoneal implants, plaque lesions, and adhesions; and it has limited field of view. TRUS is a very important and sensitive modality for POD/deep rectovaginal nodule—highly sensitive/specific for rectal endometriosis and is superior to MRI (97%/89%).

The purpose of imaging in DIE is twofolds—first is diagnosis and the extent of the lesion and second is actual preoperative mapping, which helps in planning of surgery and counseling of patients. When doing the scanning, one must look for following information:

- Size of the lesion
- Extent of depth of invasion
- Distance from anal verge
- Percentage of intestinal lumen involved
- Presence of multifocal DIE lesions.

### Transvaginal Sonography

Transvaginal sonography is the primary tool for noninvasive preoperative evaluation of DIE and bowel endometriosis and its usefulness has been highlighted in various studies. It is also observed that addition of 3D TVS may not increase the sensitivity of 2D TVS in diagnosis significantly, though it may help in demarcation and mapping of the extent of lesion.[22,23] Intestinal DIE is usually seen as a hypoechoic, round lesion within the intestinal wall with poorly delimited margins.

### Transrectal Ultrasonography

Transrectal ultrasonography with high-frequency probes, though underused, provides a reliable means to diagnose any infiltration of the bowel wall and is recommended as modality of choice for diagnosing endometriosis of deep-seated origin such as rectal, rectovaginal, uterosacral, or rectosigmoid areas.[24] It has high sensitivity and specificity for diagnosing bowel wall infiltration, better than MR imaging.

### Magnetic Resonance Imaging

Magnetic resonance imaging is another tool, which is indispensable especially in suspected cases of deep infiltrative endometriosis involving rectovaginal or bladder endometriosis. It offers a wide field of view, less operator dependence, and offers advantage in adolescent patients. It also provides an added advantage of making a complete visualization of both anterior and posterior compartments of the pelvis at same time. Sensitivity of MRI can be improved by addition of phased array coils, endovaginal coils, and rectal-contrast enema.

## MANAGEMENT (FIGS. 1 TO 4)

There is no fixed protocol for treatment in DIE and most of the time, it depends on the presenting symptoms, individual requirement, as well as severity of disease. Surgery remains the mainstay of treatment, as these cases do not respond to medical treatment most of the time and laparoscopic approach is the gold standard and preferred modality.

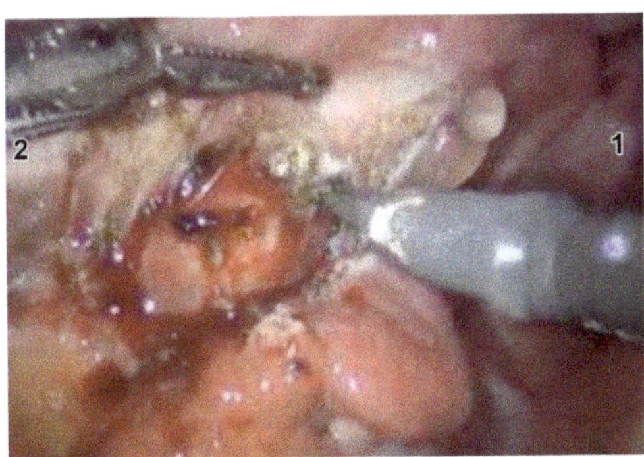

**Fig. 1:** Rectovaginal endometriosis—laparoscopic resection.

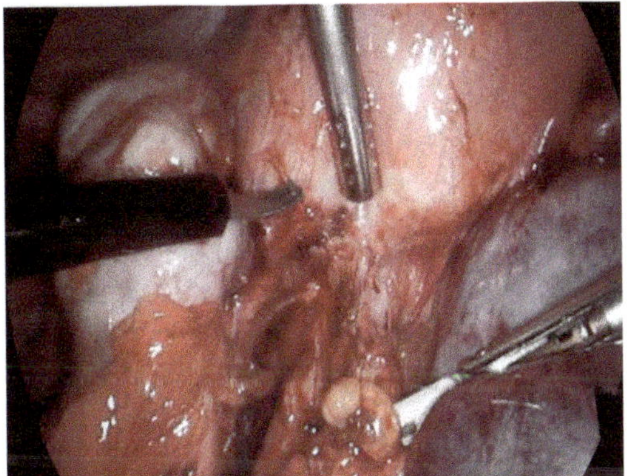

**Fig. 2:** Rectovaginal nodular dissection.

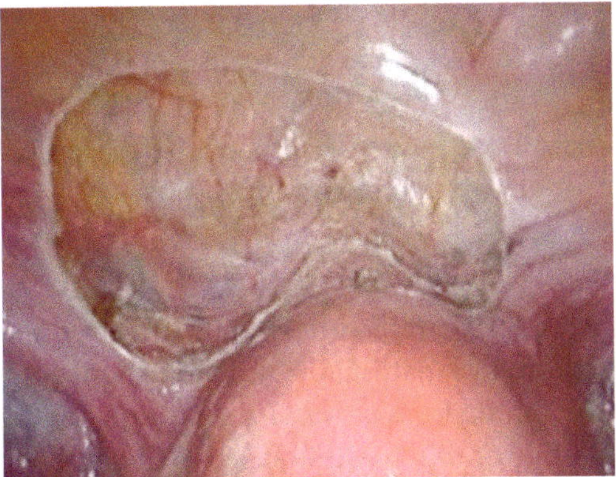

**Fig. 3:** Bladder endometriosis.

Recurrence rate is high, if surgery is not complete; so, it is recommended that all visible lesions should be excised even if it requires an extensive dissection. One should follow a targeted approach for dissection as per location of lesion as per classification.

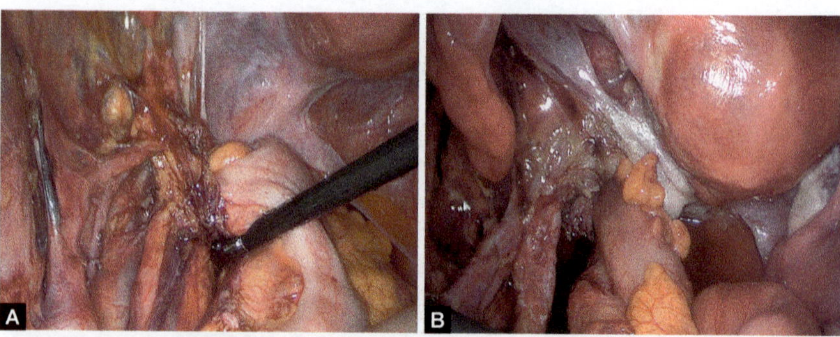

**Figs. 4A and B:** Ureterolysis.

**Table 2:** Deeply infiltrating endometriosis (DIE) classification: proposition for surgical procedure.

| DIE classification | Operative procedure |
| --- | --- |
| *A: Anterior DIE* | |
| A1: Bladder | Laparoscopic partial cystectomy |
| *P: Posterior DIE* | |
| P1: Uterosacral ligament | Laparoscopic resection of USL |
| P2: Vagina | Laparoscopic-assisted vaginal resection of DIE infiltrating posterior fornix |
| P3: Intestine | |
| Solely intestinal | |
| Without vaginal infiltration (V–) | Intestinal resection by laparoscopy/laparotomy |
| With vaginal infiltration (V+) | Laparoscopic-assisted vaginal intestinal resection or exeresis by laparotomy |
| Multiple intestinal location | Intestinal resection by laparotomy |

**Table 2** enlists the broad outlines of procedures recommended for specific type of lesion; however, they can be combined as per individual requirement.

## Endometriosis of the Bladder

Primary goal of treatment is complete resection of involved bladder wall, which can be best carried out by laparoscopy by an experienced surgeon. Bladder is dissected and separated from cervicoisthmic junction and the infiltrated bladder wall is mobilized till a visible disease-free vesicouterine space is reached. Partial bladder resection is carried out, leaving healthy margins from all sides. The bladder is then repaired in two layers without tension. Catheter is left in situ for continuous drainage for 6 days post-surgery for perfect healing. The neurogenic bladder is the most serious complication caused by vesical denervation either because of endometriosis itself or because of extensive dissection.

## Ureteric Endometriosis

There are two types of ureteric involvement. Purpose is to free the ureter and to relieve the ureteric obstruction because of endometriosis around the ureter as in extrinsic endometriosis. Extensive ureterolysis and complete dissection of pelvic ureter from its bed may be required and should be done to release the obstruction. When there is involvement of ureteric musculature and lumen as in intrinsic variety, partial resection of ureter with end-to-end anastomosis or direct ureteric implantation into the bladder with the psoas hitch technique for tension-free anastomosis may be required depending on the site of involvement. The ureter is freed of surrounding tissue all the way to its junction with the bladder to allow safe resection of the infiltrated parametria. At the same time, the retroperitoneal course of nerves lying in the operative field (such as the hypogastric, splanchnic, femoral, and obturator nerves) must be laparoscopically freed, so that a neurogenic bladder-emptying disturbance can be avoided. After extensive surgery in the area of the ureters, it is recommended that ureteric stents should be left in place for 4–6 weeks.[18]

## Intestinal DIE

Types of intestinal DIE are:

- *Multifocal disease*: It means disease spread within 2 cm area of main DIE lesion, seen in 62% of retrieved specimens.

- *Multicentral disease*: It means lesions are present beyond 2 cm area of main lesion, present in approximately 38% of cases.[25]

### *Laparoscopic Surgical Techniques*

There are mainly two approaches depending of severity and spread of disease. Choice also depends on expertise and preference of surgeon.

Conservative approach (nodular resection) is associated with low morbidity, better digestive function, and low urinary complications but higher recurrence. It is preferred in multifocal but smaller lesions on the other hand, radical approach (segmental resection) is preferred, if lesion is more than 2 cm or occlusion is more than 50%.[26]

*Nodular excision:* Multiple techniques of nodular excision are suggested and practiced. Aim is to remove rectosigmoid nodule along with part of anterior rectal wall without compromising lumen diameter.

- *Rectal shaving:*[27-29] Only good for superficial invasion < 50%. Minimal removal of adjacent rectal wall:
  - Traditional technique
  - Reverse technique.

- *Mucosal skinning:*[30] Only the mucosa is preserved intact and the deficiency in the bowel wall muscle layer is closed with suture. If mucosa is opened during procedure, it is also closed by primary suture.
- *Full-thickness anterior rectal wall excision/disk resection:*[27,31]
    - Scissors and suture—especially for smaller nodules infiltrating deeper than the muscular layer of the bowel.
    - Circular stapler—indicated for a single intestinal DIE lesion located at the anterior rectosigmoid wall, <30 mm diameter, and affecting less than one-third of intestinal circumference. Double stapler can be used, if lesion is >30 mm.
    - Linear stapler.

### Radical Surgery

It may also be called segmental bowel resection.

This involves segmental resection of bowel with end-to-end anastomosis along with or without proximal ileostomy. This is indicated in deep, large lesions > 60 mm diameters and > 50% lumen occlusion.

Complications like leakage, dysfunction of bowel, bladder, and sexual problems are associated with surgeries of DIE and these complications are less in conservative surgery, <1%, which increases up to 30%. It has been found that the leakage rate and long-term consequences of bowel resection increase when the resection involves the lower part of the bowel. For sigmoid resection, leaks occur in <1% cases, almost without long-term problems, while for low rectal resections, leaks increase to 15% or more and carry a lifelong risk of dysfunction of bowel (30%), bladder (30%), and sexual problems (40%).[32] Therefore, it is suggested that for rectosigmoid and rectal nodules, one should attempt excision of bowel nodule; while for the sigmoid lesions, one should be more liberal with bowel resections.[26]

## CONCLUSION

Minimal invasive approach is the call of the day and recommended globally. Both nodular excision and segmental bowel resection can be offered depending on severity, spread, and expertise; however, conservative approach should be preferred if possible, as most of these patients are young and long-term complications are multifold in radical approach. Regardless of which technique is employed, one should keep in mind that endometriosis is a benign disease and that the main objective of the treatment is to improve the patient's quality-of-life.

## POINTS TO REMEMBER

- The combination of compelling clinical signs and symptoms can be used to make a presumptive nonsurgical diagnosis of endometriosis.

- TVS and TRUS protocols are highly accurate in making a nonsurgical diagnosis of DIE. Specific MRI adds to improve the sensitivity of diagnostic procedures.
- Role of medical therapy is limited to provide pain relief.
- Before surgery, it is imperative to know lesion size, depth, circumferential bowel involvement, and location (or distance from the anal verge in cases of rectosigmoid lesion) to optimize surgical outcomes.
- Conservative minimal invasive approach is preferable to avoid long-term complications; however, radical surgery may be the only solution to some of these intractable and advanced stage DIEs.

## REFERENCES


1. Walter AJ, Hentz JG, Magtibay PM, Cornella JL, Magrina JF. Endometriosis: correlation between histologic and visual findings at laparoscopy. Am J Obstet Gynecol. 2001;184(7):1407-13.
2. Donnez J, Nisolle M, Grandjean P, Gillerot S, Clerckx F. The place of GnRH agonists in the treatment of endometriosis and fibroids by advanced endoscopic techniques. Br J Obstet Gynaecol. 1992;99(Suppl 7):31-3.
3. Keckstein J, Ulrich U, Kandolf O, Wiesinger H, Wustlich M. Laparoscopic therapy of intestinal endometriosis and the ranking of drug treatment. Zentralbl Gynakol. 2003;125:259-66.
4. Fauconnier A, Chapron C. Endometriosis and pelvic pain: epidemiological evidence of the relationship and implications. Hum Reprod Update. 2005;11(6):595-606.
5. Somigliana E, Infantino M, Candiani M, Vignali M, Chiodini A, Busacca M, et al. Association rate between deep peritoneal endometriosis and other forms of the disease: pathogenetic implications. Hum Reprod. 2004;19(1):168-71.
6. Donnez J, Squifflet J, Donnez O, Jadoul P. Bladder endometriosis. In: Donnez J (Ed). Atlas of Operative Laparoscopy and Hysteroscopy. London: Informa UK Ltd.; 2007. pp. 85-91.
7. Donnez J, Jadoul P, Donnez O, Squifflet J. Laparoscopic excision of rectovaginal and retrocervical endometriotic lesions. In: Donnez J (Ed). Atlas of Operative Laparoscopy and Hysteroscopy. London: Informa UK Ltd.; 2007. pp. 63-75.
8. Cornillie FJ, Oosterlynck D, Lauweryns JM, Koninckx PR. Deeply infiltrating pelvic endometriosis: histology and clinical significance. Fertil Steril. 1990;53(6):978-83.
9. Donnez J, Nisolle M, Casanas RF, Brion P, Da Costa Ferreira N. Stereometric evaluation of peritoneal endometriosis and endometriotic nodules of the rectovaginal septum. Hum Reprod. 1996;11:224-8.
10. Bochaton Piallat ML, Gabbiani G, Hinz B. The myofibroblast in wound healing and fibrosis: answered and unanswered questions. F1000 Res. 2016;5:752-9.
11. Chapron C, Fauconnier A, Vieira M, Barakat H, Dousset B, Pansini V, et al. Anatomic distribution of deeply infiltrating endometriosis: surgical implications and proposition for a classification. Hum Reprod. 2003;18(1):157-61.
12. Chapron C, Dubuisson JB. Laparoscopic treatment of deep endometriosis located on the uterosacral ligaments. Hum Reprod. 1996;11(4):868-73.
13. Kamina P. Anatomie GyneÂcologiquee tobsteÂtricale. 4. Paris: Maloine SA; 1984. p. 298.
14. Martin DC, Batt RE. Retrocervical, retrovaginal pouch, and rectovaginal septum endometriosis. J Am Assoc Gynecol Laparosc. 2001;8(1):12-7.

15. Vercellini P, Trespidi L, De Giorgi O, Cortesi I, Parazzini F, Crosignani PG. Endometriosis and pelvic pain: relation to disease stage and localisation. Fertil Steril. 1996;65(2):299-304.

16. Garry R. Laparoscopic excision of endometriosis: the treatment of choice. Br J Obstet Gynaecol. 1997;104:513-5.

17. Donnez J, Squifflet J. Laparoscopic excision of deep endometriosis. Obstet Gynecol Clin North Am. 2004;31:567-80.

18. Pérez-Utrilla Pérez M, Aguilera Bazán A, Alonso Dorrego JM, Hernández A, de Francisco MG, Martín Hernández M, et al. Urinary tract endometriosis: clinical, diagnostic, and therapeutic aspects. Urology. 2009;73(1):47-51.

19. Howard WJ, John AR. Endometriosis. Te Linde's Operative Gynecology, 11th edition. Philadelphia: Wolters Kluwer; 2014. pp. 403-45.

20. Hudelist G, Tuttlies F, Rauter G, Pucher S. Can transvaginal sonography predict infiltration depth in patients with deep infiltrating endometriosis of the rectum? Human Reprod. 2009;24(5):1012-7.

21. ESHRE Endometriosis Guideline Development Group. Guidelines of the European Society of Human Reproduction and Embryology. 2013.

22. Grasso RF, di Giacomo B, Sedati P, Sizzi O, Florio G, Faiella E, et al. Diagnosis of deep infiltrating endometriosis: accuracy of magnetic resonance imaging and transvaginal 3D ultrasonography. Abdom Imag. 2010;35(6):716-25.

23. Guerriero S, Alcazar JL, Ajossa S, Pilloni M, Melis GB. Three-dimensional sonographic characteristics of deep endometriosis. J Ultrasound Med. 2009;28(8):1061-6.

24. Chapron C, Dubuisson JB. Management of deep endometriosis. Ann NY Acad Sci. 2001;943:276-80.

25. Kavallaris A, Kohler C, Kuhne-Heid R, Schneider A. Histopathological extent of rectal invasion by rectovaginal endometriosis. Hum Reprod. 2003;18(6):1323-7.

26. Koninckx PR, Meuleman C, Oosterlynck D, Cornillie FJ. Diagnosis of deep endometriosis by clinical examination during menstruation and plasma CA-125 concentration. Fertil Steril. 1996;65(2):280-7.

27. Kondo W, Zomer MT, Ribeiro R, Trippia C, Oliveira MAP. Surgical treatment of intestinal deep infiltrating endometriosis by laparoscopy—technical aspects.

28. Kondo W, Bourdel N, Jardon K, Tamburro S, Cavoli D, Matsuzaki S, et al. Comparison between standard and reverse laparoscopic techniques for rectovaginal endometriosis. Surg Endosc. 2011;25(8):2711-7.

29. Donnez J, Squifflet J. Complications, pregnancy and recurrence in a prospective series of 500 patients operated on by the shaving technique for deep rectovaginal endometriotic nodules. Hum Reprod. 2010;25(8):1949-58.

30. Koninckx PR, Ussia A, Adamyan L, Wattiez A, Donnez J. Deep endometriosis: definition, diagnosis, and treatment. Fertil Steril. 2012;98(3):564-71.

31. Crispi CP, Schor E, Oliveira MAP, Abraão M, Ribeiro PAAG. Treaty of Gynecological Endoscopy: Cirurgia Minimally Invasive, 3rd edition. Rio de Janeiro: Revinter; 2012.

32. Ret Davalos ML, De Cicco C, D'Hoore A, De DB, Koninckx PR. Outcome after rectum or sigmoid resection: a review for gynecologists. J Minim Invasive Gynecol. 2007;14(1):33-8.

# Recent Consensus in Management of Endometriosis

*T Ramani Devi, N Gayathri*

## INTRODUCTION

Endometriosis is defined as the presence of extrauterine estrogen sensitive, progesterone-resistant endometrial-like tissue which roughly affects 10–15% of all reproductive age women. According to the researcher Merli Saare, nobody actually knows exactly how many women are being affected by this disease because there is no method for identifying endometriosis from blood sample. Today the disease is mainly diagnosed radiologically and surgically. According to the World Endometriosis Society, 176 million women are affected by endometriosis.

Endometriosis constitutes a significant burden on the quality of life of women, their families, and healthcare systems. The true prevalence rate in general population is not known mainly because the diagnosis is often overlooked by primary care doctors and it is delayed for an average of 6–9 years. Average age of diagnosis is 27 years. Generally, 30–50% of women with endometriosis are infertile (Bulletti C, et al.). Among the overall Indian population, approximately 26 million women of age 18–35 years are affected by endometriosis according to the survey by the Endometriosis Society of India in 2007.[1] 5% of adolescent girls with dysmenorrhea not responding to analgesics are diagnosed to have endometriosis. 75–80% of women with chronic pelvic pain (CPP) have endometriosis. 0.8–12.5 billion Euros are spent every year according to the EndoCost study by the World Endometriosis Research Foundation toward the management of endometriosis and economical loss due to absenteeism from the work.

## THEORIES ON PATHOGENESIS OF ENDOMETRIOSIS

Theories, which explain the development of endometriosis, include retrograde menstruation (Sampson, 1925), coelomic metaplasia (Mayer, 1924; Iwanoff, 1898; Lauche, 1923), hormonal theory (Novak, 1931), apoptosis suppression and alteration (Ferryman, 1994; Taniguchi, 2011), genetics (Hadfield, 1994; Seli, 2003; Alberisen, 2013), immune dysfunction (Semino, 1995), oxidative stress and inflammation (Murphy, 1998), and stem cells (Tsuji, 2008; Kato, 2012; Deane, 2013). There is no single universally accepted theory for the pathogenesis of endometriosis. It is evident that the presence of endometrial-like tissue outside the uterus causes chronic inflammatory reaction.

There is some polygenetic, polyepigenetic mechanism in the development of endometriosis.[2] Endometriosis is a hereditary and heterogeneous disease with many biochemical changes which are clonal in origin. The set of genetic and epigenetic mechanisms are transmitted at birth. This explains the hereditary aspects of the predisposition and endometriosis-associated changes in the endometrium, immunology, and placentation. Female fetuses who have neonatal vaginal bleeding are likely to develop endometriosis (Ivo Brosens, et al.).

## EPIDEMIOLOGICAL FACTORS AND MOLECULAR MECHANISMS INVOLVED IN ENDOMETRIOSIS DEVELOPMENT

Previous researchers have shown that endometriosis is prevalent after menarche (at the onset of thelarche) and dramatically decreases after menopause, which has led them to believe that the disorder is estrogen dependent.

Various epidemiological factors, which drastically influence the development of endometriosis, include early menarche, short menstrual cycle, increased duration of menstrual flow, and decreased parity.

Other constitutional factors include a positive family history (6.9 times higher incidence), alcohol drinking, sedentary lifestyle, and inconsistent diet. Smoking has got no effect.

## MOLECULAR AND CELLULAR ALTERATIONS

There is altered steroid biosynthesis and receptor response, which includes increased estrogen receptor $\beta$ (ER$\beta$) expression, increased aromatase expression, and perturbations in progesterone signal intermediates: HOXA10, FOXA1, NF-kB, Hic-5, NCOR2, and 17$\beta$-hydroxysteroid dehydrogenase 2 deficiencies.

Increased peritoneal vascular endothelial growth factor (VEGF), overactive AKT, upregulated matrix metalloproteinase (MMP) expression, and recruitment of Tie-2 expressing macrophages are few factors which contribute to increased invasiveness and vascularization. Certain other inflammatory responses, which trigger endometriosis, include production of chemokines such as interleukin-8 (IL-8), monocyte chemoattractant protein-1 (MCP-1), RANTES, peritoneal IL-6, and tumor necrosis factor-$\alpha$ (TNF-$\alpha$), recruitment of alternatively activated macrophages, engagement of NF-kB dependent pathway, and accumulation of iron and reactive oxygen species (ROS) production.[3]

## ETIOPATHOGENESIS

The widely accepted hypothesis is that there is retrograde spill of endometrial cells into the peritoneal cavity which gets adherent to the peritoneal surface and invades under the influence of MMP. They grow under the influence of estrogens, VEGF, and nerve growth factor (NGF). There are lots of proinflammatory factors which promote the growth of endometriosis like IL, cytokines, etc. The transmigration of the cells via lymphatics and vascular channels can explain the presence of endometriosis in remote places.

## PROGESTERONE RECEPTOR CHANGES IN ENDOMETRIOSIS (FIG. 1)

In a healthy endometrium under the influence of progesterone, cellular proliferation, decidualization, and apoptosis occur in a sequential manner. Progesterone has got anti-inflammatory and antiangiogenic effects whereas in endometriosis, there is progesterone resistant, which influences both eutopic and ectopic endometrium leading to increased cellular proliferation, impaired decidualization, and reduced apoptosis. Progesterone resistance also causes proinflammation.

Sensory nerve proliferation, activation, and neurogenic inflammation via nociceptive signaling lead to severe pain. This can also be activated through entrapment of nerve fibers during the severe stages of endometriosis.[4]

## AIM OF THE TREATMENT

According to the American Society for Reproductive Medicine (ASRM)—"endometriosis should be viewed as a chronic inflammatory disease (which is estrogen dependent and progesterone resistant) that requires a lifelong management plan with the goal of maximizing the use of medical treatment and avoiding repeated surgical procedures".

The focus of the treatment depends upon the age, fertility requirements, symptoms, severity, pretreatment, cost involved, side effects of the treatment,

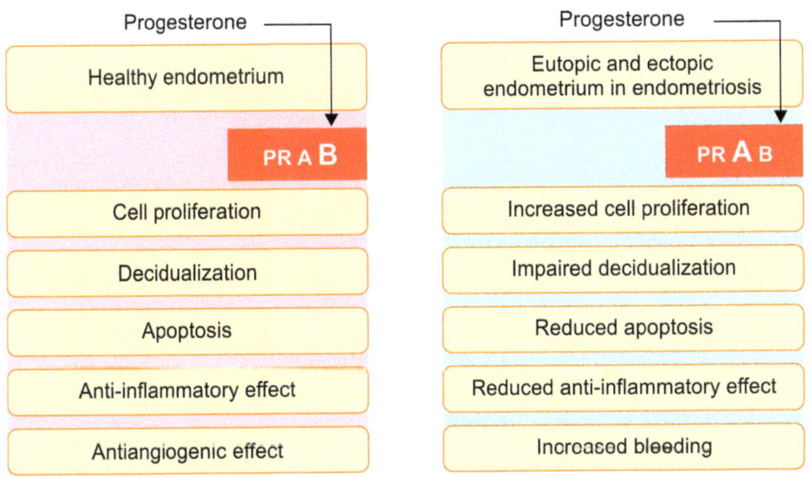


**Fig. 1:** Progesterone receptor changes in endometriosis.

and finally evidence based. Aim of the treatment includes pain relief, promoting fertility, and preventing recurrence.[5]

## TREATMENT OF ENDOMETRIOSIS

Basically, the treatment of endometriosis is either medical or surgical. The surgical management focuses on removing the lesions and regaining the pelvic anatomy. The main aim of the medical treatment is to destroy and prevent the recurrence of lesion. The surgical management should always be followed by medical management because 20% of the patients have recurrence at the end of 2 years and 50% of the patients have recurrence at the end of 5 years following surgery.[6]

### Currently Available Medical Treatments (Table 1)

- Nonsteroidal anti-inflammatory drugs (NSAIDs)
- Oral pills
- Gonadotropin-releasing hormone (GnRH) agonist
- *Progesterone*:
  - Lynestrenol
  - Gestrinone
  - Medroxyprogesterone acetate (MPA)
  - Norethisterone
- Danazol.

There are limitations to currently available medical therapy.[7]

Nonsteroidal anti-inflammatory drugs often are considered for pain management. For women who desire to conceive, COX-1 inhibitors should

**Table 1:** Currently available medical treatments.

| | |
|---|---|
| NSAIDs | Nausea, vomiting, gastrointestinal irritation, drowsiness, headache |
| Combined oral contraceptives | Nausea, weight gain, fluid retention, depression, breakthrough bleeding, breast tenderness, headache, decreased menstrual flow |
| Progestins | Nausea, weight gain, fluid retention, breakthrough bleeding, depression, amenorrhea, delayed return of ovulation |
| GnRH agonists | Hypoestrogenism (vasomotor symptoms, vaginal dryness, decreased libido, irritability, loss of bone mineral density). It has mainly central action and minimal peripheral action |
| Danazol | Hyperandrogenic side effects (acne, edema, decreased breast size) |

(GnRH: gonadotropin-releasing hormone; NSAIDs: nonsteroidal anti-inflammatory drugs)
*Source*: Giudice LC. Endometriosis. N Engl J Med. 2010;362(25):2389-98.

be considered since COX-2 inhibitors affect ovulation. NSAIDs provide only pain relief and there is no effect upon endometriosis.

Oral contraceptive pills (OCPs) often are administrated as continuous therapy rather than cyclical use and they provide slightly better pain management. However, while using these drugs in the long run, associated risks have to be remembered which include increased risk of venous thromboembolism (VTE) and effect upon fertility as they cause amenorrhea. According to Prof Chapron, young girls who consume OCPs for dysmenorrhea are likely to have deeply infiltrative endometriotic lesions.[8] Vercellini et al.[3] also quote that estrogen component of OCP will prevent the apoptosis of the shedding endometrial cells and rescue them which are something like adding fuel to the fire. Women > 35 years, history of smoking, previous myocardial infarction, thromboembolic events, stroke, etc., cannot be advised OCPs.

Next option is monotherapy with progestins which blocks MMPs, which suppresses angiogenesis and growth factors like VEGF and epidermal growth factor (EGF). Progesterone suppresses peripheral estrogen and inflammatory reactions providing symptomatic relief **(Fig. 2)**. The only side effect of progestin monotherapy is breakthrough bleeding and when used for long-term, it may cause bone mineral density (BMD) loss, if add-back therapy is not given.

## DIENOGEST (FIG. 3)

Another striking innovation in endometriosis management is dienogest which is the only progestin that combines the properties of both 19-nor-progestin

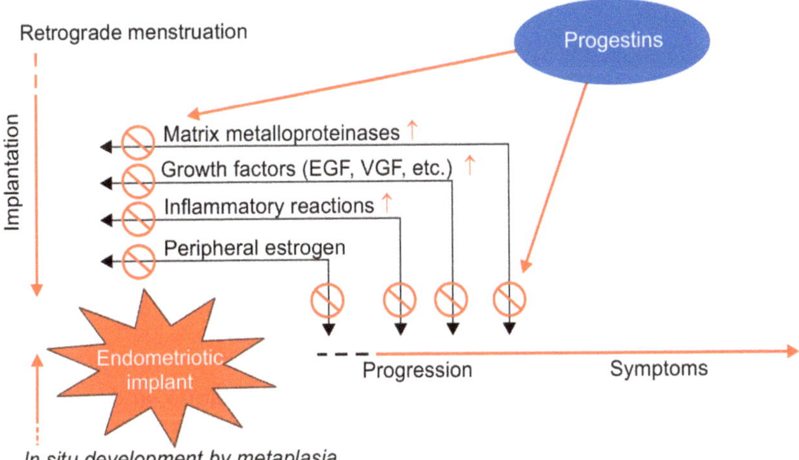


**Fig. 2:** Mechanism of retrograde menstruation.
(EGF: epidermal growth factor; VGF: vascular growth factor)
*Source:* Schweppe KW. The current place of progestins in the treatment of endometriosis. Exp Rev Obstet Gynecol. 2012;7(2):141-8.

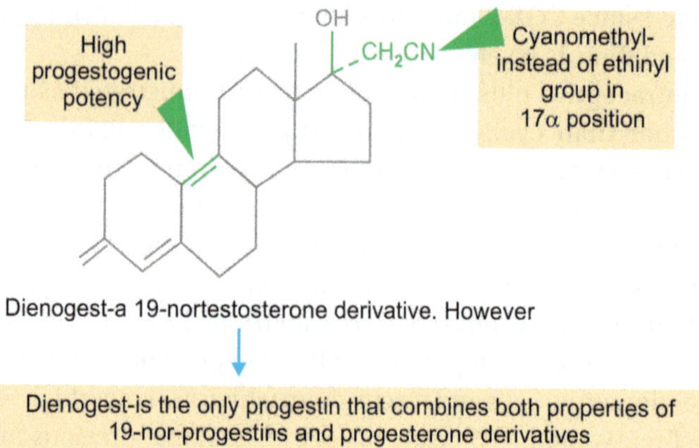



**Fig. 3:** Structure of Dienogest.

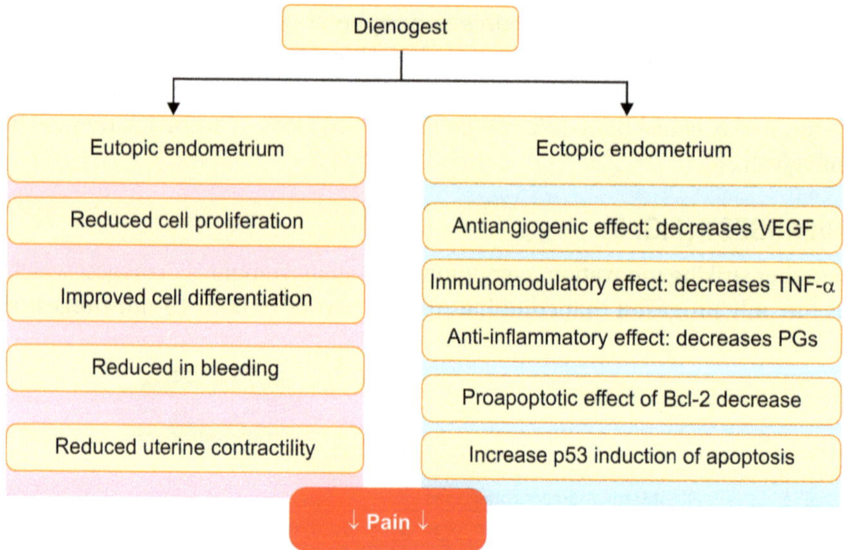



**Fig. 4:** Eutopic endometrium versus ectopic endometrium.
(PGs: prostaglandins; TNF-α: tumor necrosis factor-α; VEGF: vascular endothelial growth factor)

and progesterone derivatives. Dienogest acts in eutopic endometrium by decreasing cell proliferation, improving cell differentiation, and decreasing bleeding and uterine contractions. In ectopic endometrium, it exhibits antiangiogenic effect by decreasing VEGF, provides immune modulatory effects by decreasing TNF-α, anti-inflammatory effect by decreasing the prostaglandins, by decreasing the proapoptotic effect of Bcl-2, and triggering p53-induced apoptosis leading to reduction of pain **(Fig. 4)**.

## Indications for Dienogest

Dienogest can be safely administrated to adolescents. Dienogest can be used for endometriomas, prevention of recurrence after surgery, extragenital endometriosis (bladder, colon, and scar), adenomyosis, and prior to in vitro fertilization (IVF).

Dienogest is used at the dosage of 2 mg/day which reduces 70–80% of the endometriosis-associated pelvic pain (EAPP). Studies have shown that dienogest can also be used for a long-term.[8-10]

Dienogest versus placebo trial for a period of 12 weeks shows that the former reduces the visual analog scale (VAS) score of EAPP.[11]

Randomized multicentric open label trial over a period of 24 weeks shows that dienogest is as effective as leuprolide acetate with minimal side effects and offers good safety profile and tolerability. The problem of the breakthrough bleeding with dienogest can be overcome by prior use of leuprolide depot for a period of 3 months.[12]

## Visanne Study to Assess Safety in Adolescents Study

This study was approved by the Paediatric Committee [postoperative cognitive dysfunction (POCD)] of the European Medicines Agency (EMA) among adolescent girls. It is a multicentric single arm open label study conducted in 21 centers in six European countries during the period of March 2011 to June 2014. About 111 adolescent girls aged 12–18 years with suspicion or proven endometriosis were included in the study. The study duration was 52 weeks and follow-up was done every month. All the patients were given 2 mg of dienogest.[13]

About 78% of the adolescent girls were free of symptoms at the end of 52 weeks where the VAS score has decreased from 70 to 9 mm.[13] 84% of the adolescent girls were very much satisfied at the end of treatment. Side effects are minimal reduction in BMD, breakthrough bleeding, breast discomfort, depression, nausea, acne, and weight gain which is seen in less than 5% of the adolescent girls.

Bone mineral density reduction is not severe as dienogest maintains the estrogen threshold levels unlike GnRH agonists.

## MANAGEMENT OF ENDOMETRIOSIS IN ADULTS

Women with endometrioma not desirous of fertility can be maintained on oral dienogest for a long-term.[14] Return of fertility is much earlier when compared to GnRH analogs.

Recurrence of endometriosis either in the form of symptom recurrence or lesion recurrence can also be managed medically with dienogest.[15]

Dienogest is a novel conservative alternative to surgery for extragenital endometriosis like *deeply infiltrating endometriosis* (DIE), bladder

**Table 2:** Postoperative treatment options versus recurrence period after treatment.

| Postoperative treatment options and duration* Recurrence period after treatment* | No medication[5] | GnRH[2,6,7] | OC[1] | | Vitamin[3,4] | |
|---|---|---|---|---|---|---|
| | N/A | 6 months | <1 year | >1 year | 6 months | 5 years |
| 18 months | n/a | 10.3% | n/a | n/a | n/a | n/a |
| 2 years | 21.5% | n/a | n/a | n/a | 4% | n/a |
| 3 years | n/a | 12.8% | 49% | 22% | n/a | n/a |
| 4 years | n/a | n/a | n/a | n/a | 21% | n/a |
| 5 years | Up to 50% | 53.4% | n/a | n/a | n/a | 2.6% |

Long-term treatment is suggested
Medication after operation reduces recurrences rate
(GnRH: gonadotropin-releasing hormone; OC: oral contraceptive)

endometriosis, and scar endometriosis.[16] Symptoms are dramatically relieved with dienogest in these cases without reducing the volume of DIE.[17,18] Regarding scar endometriosis, presurgical use of dienogest may reduce the size of the lesion thereby aiding in surgical correction.

Vercellini et al. study shows the recurrence rate after treatment with dienogest is 2.6% at the end of 5 years versus GnRH analogs which are 53.4% **(Table 2)**.[6,19-22]

Hence, postsurgical patients can be maintained on long-term management with dienogest for prevention of recurrence (both pain and lesion recurrence).[23]

## Gonadotropin-releasing Hormone Agonists

Gonadotropin-releasing hormone agonists like leuprolide, goserelin, and triptorelin are used in the medical management of endometriosis as per the European Society of Human Reproduction and Embryology (ESHRE) guidelines and the *Federation of Obstetrics and Gynaecological Societies of India-Good Clinical Practice Recommendations* (FOGSI-GCPR). GnRH analog is the first-line drug with level A evidence. The mechanism of action is both at central and peripheral. It downregulates the hypothalamic-pituitary-ovarian (HPO) axis and hence estradiol (E2) production is lowered by the ovaries. This suppresses the endometriotic tissue. The peripheral action is mild.

Main disadvantages of GnRH agonists are that it cannot be used beyond 6 months as per the Food and Drug Administration (FDA). Beyond 3 months, add-back therapy is a must. It causes BMD reduction, hot flushes, dryness of vagina, headache, depression, mood swings, and loss of libido.[24,25]

Recurrence of endometriosis in the postoperative period is reduced only when six doses are used (ESHRE, 2014). At the end of 5 years follow-up postoperatively, the recurrence incidence is up to 53% comparable to no treatment.[6] But prior to assisted reproductive technology (ART), three doses of GnRH agonists improve pregnancy outcome by fourfold.[26]

## Dydrogesterone

It can be administered as 10 mg twice daily from D5 to D25 which causes atrophy of ectopic endometrium and inhibits development of newer implants. It has no effect upon the eutopic endometrium and will not inhibit ovulation. By the virtue of immunomodulatory effect, it decreases IL-1, -6, -8 and increases nitric oxide (NO) production and exhibits anti-inflammatory action. There is no weight gain or edema in these patients. It effectively relieves dysmenorrhea, dyspareunia, and pelvic pain without affecting fertility.[27] This also promotes fertility.

## Levonorgestrel-releasing Intrauterine System

Levonorgestrel-releasing intrauterine system (LNG-IUS) releases 20 µg/24 h with a lifetime of 5 years. This drug causes endometrial atrophy by continuous release within the endometrium. A very small proportion of LNG is released in peritoneal fluid which causes regression of peritoneal endometriosis. Postoperative treatment with LNG-IUS reduces pain and lesion recurrence. LNG-IUS is as effective as depot MPA (DMPA) for 3 years. Hence, it can be used safely in women following surgery for endometriosis who are not keen on conception. Most of the endometriosis patients have associated adenomyosis and LNG-IUS is the best option for these patients. LNG-IUS reduces both cyclical and noncyclical pain in endometriosis patients.[28,29]

## Danazol

Danazol is a synthetic derivative of $17\alpha$-ethinyl testosterone which suppresses luteinizing hormone (LH) surge and other ovarian enzymes responsible for steroidogenesis, which leads to hypoestrogenic and hyperandrogenic state that decreases endometrial-like tissue growth. Danazol is the first FDA approved drug for endometriosis. Due to the androgenic side effects, the drug is not used now. Still danazol-containing vaginal ring can be used in the treatment of endometriosis (particularly for DIE), pregnancy is possible with ring usage. Danazol containing intrauterine device (IUD) is used in the treatment of endometriosis who are not keen on pregnancy. When inserted within 7 days of last menstruation period (LMP), it reduces EAPP. It can be used for 6 months. Side effects include weight gain, acne, abnormal lipid profile, atrophic vaginitis, liver dysfunction, depression, hot flushes, etc.[30]

## Depot Medroxyprogesterone Acetate

Injectable DMPA subcutaneous (SC) 104 mg/DMPA intramuscular (IM) 150 mg is also equally effective in treatment of EAPP. The efficacy is comparable to that of danazol, GnRH analogs, and continuous OCPs. Main side effect is marked reduction in BMD, breakthrough bleeding, and long time taken to regain ovulation. The main advantage is cost factor.[31]

## Gonadotropin-releasing Hormone Antagonists

Gonadotropin-releasing hormone antagonists suppresses HPO axis and maintains estrogen threshold. Phase 1, 2, and 3 trials are with elagolix, abarelix, and cetrorelix show that it provides good tolerance and efficacy without postmenopausal symptoms. There is no flare effect and need for add-back therapy. Hence, it is better than GnRH agonist. Degarelix is a long-acting orally available decapeptide which can be used in the treatment of EAPP. Cetrorelix 3 mg weekly once for 8 weeks gives pain relief and regression of the lesions.[32,33]

### Elagolix

Elagolix is a recently FDA approved (July 2018) oral GnRH antagonist used for EAPP. Elagolix dose dependently decreases the estrogen levels. It is available in 150 mg or 200 mg formulations and can be used for a minimum of 6 months to a maximum of 24 months. BMD reduction occurs only with higher doses and when administered for a longer duration. So, add-back therapy is not required for short-term use. Contraindications include concomitant administration of statins, severe hepatic impairment, and osteoporosis. Elagolix is affected by estrogen-containing contraceptive methods and so nonhormonal contraception should be considered. Human studies with on cetrorelix, TAK-385, relugolix, KLH-2109, OBE-2109, and ASP-1707 are ongoing for treatment of endometriosis. Only elagolix has been FDA approved for treating endometriosis so far.[34]

## Aromatase Inhibitors

Aromatase inhibitors (AIs) have central, peripheral, and local action. It is considered as second-line drug for endometriosis. Use of AI is restricted mainly due to hot flushes. Third-generation AI like letrozole, anastrozole are potent in managing EAPP not responding to hormones and GnRH analogs. Letrozole 2.5 mg with norethisterone 5 mg when given for 6 months reduces revised American Fertility Society (rAFS) score and pain score.

Anastrozole 1 mg with 200 mg micronized progesterone can be given for 6 months. GnRH analogs and anastrozole improve pain management than GnRHa alone. Typically, AIs are used off-label for refractory severe endometriosis and are often given in combination with progestins because AIs alone causes reduction in BMD and increased follicle-stimulating hormone (FSH) which results in ovarian cysts.[24]

Third-generation AIs are reversible, potent with faster pharmacokinetics.

## Selective Estrogen Receptor Modulators

Selective estrogen receptor modulators (SERMs)—tamoxifen and raloxifene at a dose of 10 mg/kg provide antiproliferative effect on endometrium by causing regression of implants in 40–50% of patients. SERM provides beneficial estrogen effects on bone mineralization without stimulating the endometrium or breasts. Raloxifene is effective for postmenopausal osteoporosis, but women under raloxifene had more pelvic pain and required additional surgical correction.

One-third generation of SERM is bazedoxifene which blocks the ER selectively in endometrium without affecting bone or central nervous system (CNS).[35] It regresses the endometriotic lesions. Bazedoxifene with conjugated estrogens is the first tissue selective estrogen complex which was FDA approved drug for symptomatic menopause treatment. It fully resolves EAPP along with continued ovulation.

Side effects are hot flushes, VTE, diarrhea, neck pain, spasms, etc.

## Selective Progesterone Receptor Modulators

Selective progesterone receptor modulators (SPRMs) are progesterone receptor ligands with high degree of endometriosis selectivity. These drugs (mainly asoprisnil) inhibit endometrial proliferation and suppress prostaglandin production with estrogen deprivation.[36] Even when given in minimal doses, it reduces dysmenorrhea. So far, it is safe and its tolerability is good with no reported adverse effects.

Progesterone antagonists (mifepristone and onapristone) modulate progesterone receptors in ectopic and eutopic endometrium. With dose of 25 mg, it reduces pain and 50 mg reduces the size of lesion. It also exhibits antiglucocorticoid property.

RU-485 in 5, 25, and 50 mg can be given for 6 months.

Major drawback is that it may lead to hypoadrenalism.

Mifepristone exerts dose-dependent progesterone antagonistic effect to suppress endometrial growth and blood supply.

A recent Cochrane review stated that mifepristone improved dysmenorrhea in endometriosis in majority of patients whereas dyspareunia was reduced only in a minority of patients.[36]

Tanaproget is a new SPRM which suppresses MMP expression on endometrial cells. However, there are only limited in vitro studies in human and mice model to support its role in endometriosis.[37]

## Estrogen Receptor Ligands

Estrogen receptor ligands called selective estrogen receptor-beta agonists are highly selective in ERβ binding more than ERα binding. Drugs included are oxabicycloheptene sulfonate and chloroindazole. They provide anti-inflammatory and antiproliferative effects. Human studies are ongoing with phase II trial. This drug does not prevent pregnancy.[38]

## Antiangiogenic Drugs

As endometriotic lesions demand vascular support for growth and produce VEGE, angiogenic inhibitors belong to a new category in treatment of endometriosis. Previous animal studies (but not yet in humans) are available with TNP-470 (lodamin, endostatin, avastin, anginex, romidepsin, etc.).[24]

Here statins suppress MMPs and provide anti-inflammatory, antiangiogenic, and antioxidant properties in addition to correcting hyperlipidemia. Single trial with atorvastatin 20 mg/day for 6 months with OCPs is available.

Dopamine receptor 2 agonists that cause VEGF-2 dephosphorylation include cabergoline and quinagolide. A significant lower proliferation index is observed with cabergoline and also decreases neoangiogenesis. Cabergoline is more effective than GnRH agonist in reducing endometrioma size.[39] Cabergoline also reduces pain by acting through nerve fibers. It is used in early stages of disease and DIE. It also normalizes menstrual cycles, prevents progression of endometriosis, and reduces the recurrence rates.

In addition, studies have demonstrated some success where cabergoline is used for reducing endometriotic lesion other than its effect in correction of hyperprolactinemia. Quinagolide is used for treatment of endometriosis-associated hyperprolactinemia. By exhibiting fibrinolytic, antiangiogenic, and anti-inflammatory effects, 35% showed vanishing of peritoneal lesions and 70% showed regression of endometriotic lesions.[40]

## Rapamycin

Rapamycin also showed decrease in lesion size in a recently conducted mice trial. Rapamycin showed effect on serum levels of hypoxia-inducible factor-1α (HIF-1α) and VEGF. Rapamycin not only significantly decreased the size of the lesion but also inhibits *microvessel density* (MVD) and VEGF expression. Rapamycin is the first identified specific mammalian target of rapamycin (mTOR) inhibitor. In addition, it has antiangiogenic activity.[41]

## Immunomodulators

It includes TNF-α blockers (where proinflammatory cytokines are blocked). These drugs alter immune function and play major role in endometriosis genesis like acting on elevated cytokine levels and decreased cell apoptosis. They are mainly used in early stage endometriosis. Typical side effects include headache, allergy, reactivation of tuberculosis (TB), etc. Yet the use of TNF-α blockers for pain management is not supported by adequate evidence.

Loxoribine stimulates natural killer (NK) cell activity. TNF-α blockers prevent TNF-α release from macrophages. Pentoxifylline is currently used for intermittent claudication through competitive nonselective suppression of phosphodiesterase enzyme and anti-inflammatory action. Due to limited human studies, it continues to provide inadequate information for prescribing in treatment of endometriosis.[24]

Other drugs of peroxisome proliferator-activated receptor γ (PPARγ) ligands like rosiglitazone and pioglitazone are also under trial. They exhibit antiangiogenic and anti-inflammatory effects.

## Resveratrol

Phytotherapeutic agent resveratrol trans 3,5,4'-trihydroxystilbene found in red wine, grapes, and berries acts as pleiotropic agents. It reduces proliferation, vascularization, and free radical oxygen formation and promotes apoptosis. Its dose dependency reduces or stops angiogenesis. Resveratrol represents a promising therapy in future for treatment of endometriosis.

## Gabapentin

Neurontin (gabapentin) by suppressing spinal pain pathway is an effective treatment for CPP. But they are still under study.

Nerve growth factor has shown to be a major neurotrophic factor in endometriosis-associated pain. There is also increase in local nerve density. Further research into signaling underlying neurogenesis in endometriosis is needed to identify potential targeted treatment protocol.

## Retinoic Acid Metabolism

Recent findings suggest that retinoic acid metabolism and action are fundamentally flawed in endometriotic tissues and even genetically in women with endometriosis. Activation of retinoid signaling in endometriosis tissues is predicted to have several salutary effects on the resident cells within this lesions.[42] As a consequence of this activity in peritoneal fluid macrophages (PFMs), there is reduced inflammatory and oxidative stress of peritoneal environment and increased clearance of ectopic endometrial cells.

Recent findings include study evidence for potential development of endometriosis associated with KISS1/KISS1R system.[43]

Suppression of tumor metastasis is one among the various functions of Kisspeptides 1. Kisspeptides show some association in pathogenesis of endometriosis. Endometriosis being a progressively active disease shows some similarities with tumor process. Kisspeptins can suppress the transcription of MMP through its antimetastatic properties and possible influence in cell migration ability, invasiveness, and apoptosis.[44]

## CHINESE HERBAL MEDICINE FOR ENDOMETRIOSIS

Oral Chinese herbal medicines (CHMs) are effective in relieving dysmenorrhea and shrinking adnexal masses when used along with CHM enema but this needs more rigorous research.

Chinese herbal medicine, e.g., Yiwongn, curcuma/curcumin (found in turmeric) have found to suppress endometriotic lesions by suppressing cytokines, transcription factors, growth factor receptors, and angiogenic activity. But all these herbal medicines do not have evidence-based support for prescribing for women with endometriosis.[45]

## OTHER COMPLIMENTARY TREATMENT OF ENDOMETRIOSIS-ASSOCIATED PELVIC PAIN

Yoga and meditation can be used as adjuvant therapy. Acupuncture may be effective for severe dysmenorrhea. There is limited use of neuromodulators, behavioral therapy, reflexology, homeopathy, and psychological therapy for treatment of EAPP.

## IMPORTANT RECENT FINDINGS

In arcuate nucleus, there are neurons colocalized which comprise of three neuropeptides namely kisspeptins, neurokinin B (NKB), and dynorphin (Dyn), which are collectively known as KNDy neurons.[44]

They interact to influence the GnRH release, where kisspeptins stimulates, NKB modulates, and Dyn inhibits the pulsatile GnRH release.

Women with EAPP showed decreased gray matter volume in brain regions involved in pain perception. Women with CPP without endometriosis also showed decrease in gray matter. These changes were not seen in patients with endometriosis who had no CPP. This evidence shows that reduction in gray matter of the brain is associated with perception of pain.

## CONCLUSION

Endometriosis is a complex disease with mysterious etiology, but its origin remains obscure. Furthermore, it is responsible for both superficial and deep lesions which explain its two most well-known challenges—(1) pain and (2) infertility. The determination of blood and endometrial markers should allow a noninvasive and easily reproducible diagnosis which may be possible in future. The main aims in future are early diagnosis, replacement of invasive surgery by medical management, and preserve functions of the involved organs thereby reducing recurrence and psychological impact among suffering women. Recent work in neuroendocrinology, endocrinology, tumorigenesis, neurogenesis, and genomics markedly will change the current approach in management of endometriosis. Being a chronic inflammatory disease, it has to be managed lifelong by medical management and avoid unnecessary repeated surgical procedures.

## REFERENCES


1. India Today Web Desk (2018). Symptoms to solution: Here's all you need to know about endometriosis. [online] Available from: https://www.indiatoday.in/lifestyle/health/story/endometriosis-disorder-painful-periods-menstruation-uterus-ovaries-1199681-2018-03-28. [Last accessed March, 2020].
2. Koninckx PR, Ussia A, Adamyan L, Wattiez A, Gomel V, Martin DC. Pathogenesis of endometriosis: the genetic/epigenetic theory. Fertil Steril. 2019;111(2):327-40.
3. Vercellini P, Viganò P, Somigliana E, Fedele L. Endometriosis: pathogenesis and treatment. Nat Rev Endocrinol. 2014;10(5):261-75.
4. Laux-Biehlmann A, d'Hooghe T, Zollner TM. Menstruation pulls the trigger for inflammation and pain in endometriosis. Trends Pharmacol Sci. 2015;36(5):270-6.
5. Dalton M. Forensic Gynaecology. London: RCOG Press; 2004.
6. Guo SW. Recurrence of endometriosis and its control. Hum Reprod Update. 2009;15(4):441-61.
7. Giudice LC. Endometriosis. N Engl J Med. 2010;362(25):2389-98.
8. Chapron C, Souza C, Borghese B, Lafay-Pillet MC, Santulli P, Bijaoui G, et al. Oral contraceptives and endometriosis: the past use of oral contraceptives for treating severe primary dysmenorrhea is associated with endometriosis, especially deep infiltrating endometriosis. Hum Reprod. 2011;26(8):2028-35.
9. Römer T. Long-term treatment of endometriosis with dienogest: retrospective analysis of efficacy and safety in clinical practice. Arch Gynecol Obstet. 2018;298(4):747-53.
10. Agarwal S, Fraser MA, Chen I, Singh SS. Dienogest for the treatment of deep endometriosis: case report and literature review. J Obstet Gynaecol Res. 2015;41(2):309-13.
11. Strowitzki T, Faustmann T, Gerlinger C, Seitz C. Dienogest in the treatment of endometriosis-associated pelvic pain: a 12-week, randomized, double-blind, placebo-controlled study. Eur J Obstet Gynecol Reprod Biol. 2010;151(2):193-8.
12. Strowitzki T, Marr J, Gerlinger C, Faustmann T, Seitz C. Dienogest is as effective as leuprolide acetate in treating the painful symptoms of endometriosis: a 24-week, randomized, multicentre, open-label trial. Hum Reprod. 2010;25(3):633-41.
13. Ebert AD, Dong L, Merz M, Kirsch B, Francuski M, Böttcher B, et al. Dienogest 2 mg daily in the treatment of adolescents with clinically suspected endometriosis: the VISanne study to assess safety in ADOlescents. J Pediatr Adolesc Gynecol. 2017;30(5):560-7.
14. Sugimoto K, Nagata C, Hayashi H, Yanagida S, Okamoto A. Use of dienogest over 53 weeks for the treatment of endometriosis. J Obstet Gynaecol Res. 2015;41(12):1921-6.
15. Lee JH, Song JY, Yi KW, Lee SR, Lee DY, Shin JH, et al. Effectiveness of dienogest for treatment of recurrent endometriosis: multicenter data. Reprod Sci. 2018;25(10):1515-22.
16. Harada M, Osuga Y, Izumi G, Takamura M, Takemura Y, Hirata T, et al. Dienogest, a new conservative strategy for extragenital endometriosis: a pilot study. Gynecol Endocrinol. 2011;27(9):717-20.

17. Leonardo-Pinto JP, Benetti-Pinto CL, Cursino K, Yela DA. Dienogest and deep infiltrating endometriosis: the remission of symptoms is not related to endometriosis nodule remission. Eur J Obstet Gynecol Reprod Biol. 2017;211:108-11.

18. Yela DA, Kajikawa P, Donati L, Cursino K, Giraldo H, Benetti-Pinto CL. Deep infiltrating endometriosis treatment with dienogest: a pilot study. J Endometr Pelvic Pain Disord. 2015;7(1):33-7.

19. Vercellini P, Somigliana E, Daguati R, Vigano P, Meroni F, Crosignani PG. Postoperative oral contraceptive exposure and risk of endometrioma recurrence. Am J Obstet Gynecol. 2008;198(5):504.e1-5.

20. Yanase T, Tsuneki I, Tamura M, Kurabayashi T. Relief of uterine bleeding by cyclic administration of dienogest for endometriosis. Gynecol Endocrinol. 2014;30(11):804-7.

21. Ota Y, Andou M, Yanai S, Nakajima S, Fukuda M, Takano M, et al. Long-term administration of dienogest reduces recurrence after excision of endometrioma. J Endometr Pelvic Pain Disord. 2015;7(2):63-7.

22. Waller KG, Shaw RW. Gonadotropin-releasing hormone analogues for the treatment of endometriosis: long-term follow-up. Fertil Steril. 1993;59(3):511-5.

23. Adachi K, Takahashi K, Nakamura K, Otake A, Sasamoto N, Miyoshi Y, et al. Postoperative administration of dienogest for suppressing recurrence of disease and relieving pain in subjects with ovarian endometriomas. Gynecol Endocrinol. 2016;32(8):646-9.

24. Bedaiwy MA, Allaire C, Yong P, Alfaraj S. Medical management of endometriosis in patients with chronic pelvic pain. Semin Reprod Med. 2017;35(1):38-53.

25. Zito G, Luppi S, Giolo E, Martinelli M, Venturin I, Di Lorenzo G, et al. Medical treatments for endometriosis-associated pelvic pain. Biomed Res Int. 2014;2014:191967.

26. Sallam HN, Garcia-Velasco JA, Dias S, Arici A, Abou-Setta AM. Long-term pituitary down-regulation before in vitro fertilization (IVF) for women with endometriosis. Cochrane Database Syst Rev. 2006;(1):CD004635.

27. Schweppe KW. The place of dydrogesterone in the treatment of endometriosis and adenomyosis. Maturitas. 2009;65(Suppl 1):S23-7.

28. Wong AY, Tang LC, Chin RK. Levonorgestrel-releasing intrauterine system (Mirena) and depot medroxyprogesterone acetate (Depoprovera) as long-term maintenance therapy for patients with moderate and severe endometriosis: a randomised controlled trial. Aust NZJ Obstet Gynaecol. 2010;50(3):273-9.

29. Tekin YB, Dilbaz B, Altinbas SK, Dilbaz S. Postoperative medical treatment of chronic pelvic pain related to severe endometriosis: levonorgestrel-releasing intrauterine system versus gonadotropin-releasing hormone analogue. Fertil Steril. 2011;95(2):492-6.

30. Igarashi M, Iizuka M, Abe Y, Ibuki Y. Novel vaginal danazol ring therapy for pelvic endometriosis, in particular deeply infiltrating endometriosis. Hum Reprod. 1998;13(7):1952-6.

31. Jain J, Jakimiuk AJ, Bode FR, Ross D, Kaunitz AM. Contraceptive efficacy and safety of DMPA-SC. Contraception. 2004;70(4):269-75.

32. Struthers RS, Nicholls AJ, Grundy J, Chen T, Jimenez R, Yen SS, et al. Suppression of gonadotropins and estradiol in premenopausal women by oral administration of the nonpeptide gonadotropin-releasing hormone antagonist elagolix. J Clin Endocrinol Metab. 2009;94(2):545-51.

33. Küpker W, Felberbaum RE, Krapp M, Schill T, Malik E, Diedrich K. Use of GnRH antagonists in the treatment of endometriosis. Reprod Biomed Online. 2002;5(1):12-6.

34. Barra F, Scala C, Ferrero S. Elagolix sodium for the treatment of women with moderate to severe endometriosis-associated pain. Drugs Today (Barc). 2019;55(4):237-46.

35. Komm BS, Kharode YP, Bodine PV, Harris HA, Miller CP, Lyttle CR. Bazedoxifene acetate: a selective estrogen receptor modulator with improved selectivity. Endocrinology. 2005;146(9):3999-4008.

36. Fu J, Song H, Zhou M, Zhu H, Wang Y, Chen H, et al. Progesterone receptor modulators for endometriosis. Cochrane Database Syst Rev. 2017;(7):CD009881.

37. Bruner-Tran KL, Zhang Z, Eisenberg E, Winneker RC, Osteen KG. Down-regulation of endometrial matrix metalloproteinase-3 and -7 expression in vitro and therapeutic regression of experimental endometriosis in vivo by a novel nonsteroidal progesterone receptor agonist, tanaproget. J Clin Endocrinol Metab. 2006;91(4):1554-60.

38. Zhao Y, Chen Y, Kuang Y, Bagchi MK, Taylor RN, Katzenellenbogen JA, et al. Multiple beneficial roles of repressor of estrogen receptor activity (REA) in suppressing the progression of endometriosis. Endocrinology. 2015;157(2):900-12.

39. Hamid AM, Madkour WA, Moawad A, Elzaher MA, Roberts MP. Does cabergoline help in decreasing endometrioma size compared to LHRH agonist? A prospective randomized study. Arch Gynecol Obstet. 2014;290(4):677-82.

40. Gómez R, Abad A, Delgado F, Tamarit S, Simón C, Pellicer A. Effects of hyperprolactinemia treatment with the dopamine agonist quinagolide on endometriotic lesions in patients with endometriosis-associated hyperprolactinemia. Fertil Steril. 2011;95(3):882-8.

41. Ren XU, Wang Y, Xu G, Dai L. Effect of rapamycin on endometriosis in mice. Exp Ther Med. 2016;12(1):101-6.

42. Taylor RN, Kane MA, Sidell N. Pathogenesis of endometriosis: roles of retinoids and inflammatory pathways. Semin Reprod Med. 2015;33(4):246-56.

43. Makri A, Msaouel P, Petraki C, Milingos D, Protopapas A, Liapi A, et al. KISS1/KISS1R expression in eutopic and ectopic endometrium of women suffering from endometriosis. In Vivo. 2012;26(1):119-27.

44. Navarro VM. Interactions between kisspeptins and neurokinin B. In: Kauffman AS, Smith JT (Eds). Kisspeptin Signaling in Reproductive Biology. New York: Springer; 2013. pp. 325-47.

45. Flower A, Liu JP, Lewith G, Little P, Li Q. Chinese herbal medicine for endometriosis. Cochrane Database Syst Rev. 2012;(5):CD006568.

# CHAPTER 12

# Adenomyosis: Overcome the Old Challenges

*Sameena Chowdhury, Sharmin Abbasi*

## INTRODUCTION

The term "adenomyosis" comes from the words: adeno—gland, myo—muscle, and osis—condition. Adenomyosis is relatively common, although somewhat neglected, disorder of the female reproductive tract. Today, the term "adenomyoma" has a more restricted meaning, referring to a well-defined and circumscribed lesion localized in the myometrium. Adenomyosis is a condition in which the inner lining of the uterus (the endometrium) breaks through the muscle wall of the uterus (the myometrium). It is considered a specific entity in the PALM-COEIN (polyp; adenomyosis; leiomyoma; malignancy and hyperplasia; coagulopathy; ovulatory dysfunction; endometrial; iatrogenic; and not yet classified)-International Federation of Gynecology and Obstetrics (FIGO) classification of causes of abnormal uterine bleeding (AUB). Women affected by adenomyosis may present with AUB, dysmenorrhea, dyspareunia, or infertility, but one-third of them are asymptomatic. For many years, adenomyosis has remained a histopathological diagnosis made after hysterectomy in perimenopausal women with heavy menstrual bleeding (HMB) or pelvic pain. Over the last decade, adenomyosis has also become a condition identified in young fertile-age women due to the recent advancements in imaging techniques. Despite the improvement of diagnostic tools, the awareness of the condition is still poor. Furthermore, in some patients, adenomyosis coexists with other gynecological conditions such as endometriosis and uterine fibroids. Though adenomyosis is considered a benign (not life-threatening) condition, the frequent pain and heavy bleeding associated with it can have a negative impact on a woman's quality-of-life.

## CHANGING CONCEPTS IN ADENOMYOSIS FROM PAST TO PRESENT

- Diagnosis in early age of life due to modern imaging technique
- Adenomyosis is a common cause of subfertility
- Adenomyosis and endometriosis are different stages of the same disease (50–80%)
- Treatment options are—conservative, fertility restoration surgery.

## EPIDEMIOLOGY

There are wide variations in the incidence of adenomyosis between racial and ethnic groups and different geographic regions. It is not clear whether this is due to patient factors or differences in diagnosis. In addition, with an increasing number of hysterectomies performed as laparoscopic supracervical interventions, resulting consequently in morcellated uterine specimens, the spatial arrangement of the tissue is modified, leading to a different reference to the surface and making the histological diagnosis of adenomyosis more challenging. Finally, the likelihood of establishing the presence of adenomyosis is directly proportional to the number of tissue samples taken, with the diagnosis rate ranging from 31 to 62% in the same uterus.

## CAUSES

The cause of adenomyosis is not known; however, some theories have been formed about its origins. One theory is that the endometrial cells are somehow able to migrate and invade the normal uterine wall. Another theory is that cells in the uterine wall develop into endometrial cells. There have been many theories, including:

- *Invasive tissue growth*: Some experts believe that adenomyosis results from the direct invasion of endometrial cells from the lining of the uterus into the muscle that forms the uterine walls. Uterine incisions made during an operation such as a cesarean section (C-section) might promote the direct invasion of the endometrial cells into the wall of the uterus.
- *Developmental origins*: Other experts suspect that adenomyosis originates within the uterine muscle from endometrial tissue deposited there when the uterus first formed in the fetus.
- *Uterine inflammation related to childbirth*: Another theory suggests a link between adenomyosis and childbirth. Inflammation of the uterine lining during the postpartum period might cause a break in the normal boundary of cells that line the uterus. Surgical procedures on the uterus can have a similar effect.
- *Stem cell origins*: A recent theory proposes that bone marrow stem cells might invade the uterine muscle, causing adenomyosis.

## RISK FACTORS

### Age

Though this condition can affect women of any age, most women diagnosed with adenomyosis are in their 40 and 50 years of age. About 70–80% of women undergoing hysterectomy for adenomyosis are in their fourth and fifth decade of life. Several studies have reported a mean age over 50 years for women undergoing hysterectomy for adenomyosis.

## Pregnancy

A high percentage of women with adenomyosis are multiparous woman. Pregnancy might facilitate the formation of adenomyosis by allowing adenomyotic foci to be included in the myometrium due to the invasive nature of the trophoblast on the extension of the myometrial fiber. As pregnancy progresses, mechanical weakening of the myometrium may occur as the uterus becomes distended, with further resultant infiltration of the endometrial basalis.

## History of Uterine Surgery

Having previous surgery on the uterus, including cesarean section, uterine curettage significantly increases the risk of adenomyosis.

## Smoking

Association of smoking and adenomyosis is controversial. In smokers, the serum level of estrogen is less and adenomyosis has been suggested to be an estrogen-dependent disorder. So, it may be protective, but two studies even reported a higher rate of a history of smoking in women with adenomyosis than in controls. Thus, the association between adenomyosis and smoking deserves further investigation.

## History of Ectopic Pregnancy

Women with adenomyosis are more likely to have a history of ectopic pregnancy, since adenomyosis may be a risk factor for the development of intramural ectopic pregnancy.

## Psychiatric Disorder

This association may be due to abnormalities in prolactin dynamics. Exposure of the uterus to increased prolactin appears to be sufficient to cause histological adenomyosis and is associated with upregulation of the uterine prolactin receptor messenger ribonucleic acid (RNA).

## Anticancer Treatment

Adenomyosis is relatively rare in postmenopausal women, but a higher incidence of adenomyosis has been reported in women treated with tamoxifen for breast cancer. Tamoxifen is an antagonist of the estrogen receptor in breast tissue via its active metabolite, 4-hydroxytamoxifen.[1]

## PATHOGENESIS OF ADENOMYOSIS

Adenomyosis results from the invagination of basalis endometrium into the myometrium through an altered or interrupted junctional zone (JZ), which represents a highly specialized hormone-responsive structure located in the

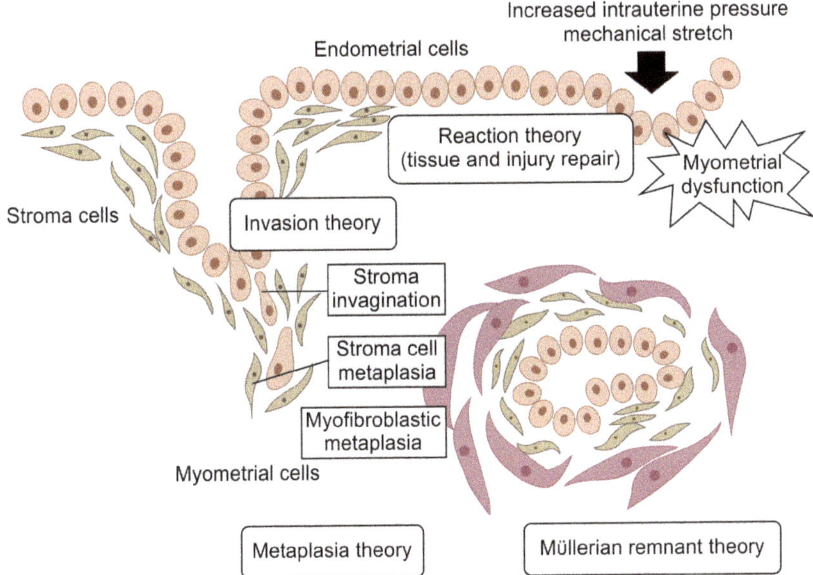


**Fig. 1:** Pathogenesis of adenomyosis.

inner third of the myometrium. As shown in **Figure 1**, molecular alterations in eutopic endometrium seem to contribute to migration and survival of ectopic endometrial implants beyond the myometrial interface. Even though alterations in apoptosis, steroid hormone responsiveness, and extracellular matrix pathways have been found in both adenomyotic lesions and eutopic endometrium, the underlying mechanisms need to be further evaluated. In addition, the role of tissue injury and repair (TIAR) as the primary mechanism for myometrial invasion has been hypothesized. Chronic peristaltic myometrial contractions may induce continuous microtrauma to the JZ, causing inflammation, which, in turn, promotes local increased estrogen production, inducing a vicious cycle.[2] A positive feedback mechanism is generated and chronic hyperperistalsis in the JZ promotes repeated cycles of autotraumatization. Invagination is commonly found on posterior wall of uterus. Invagination is also facilitated by weakness of smooth muscle tissue of uterus. Weakness may be due to high estrogen concentration in the local areal or impaired immune-related growth factor.

The question is why invasion is more commonly found on the posterior wall of the uterus. This has been found primarily on statistical basis. Moreover, in endometriosis and in adenomyosis, uterus is almost always retroverted; hence, increased intrauterine pressure is more commonly transmitted toward posterior uterine wall. Thus, the TIAR theory, stressing the importance of tissue damage to the endometrial–myometrial interface, supports the common understanding that adenomyosis is associated with multiparity, previous cesarean section, and prior uterine surgery.

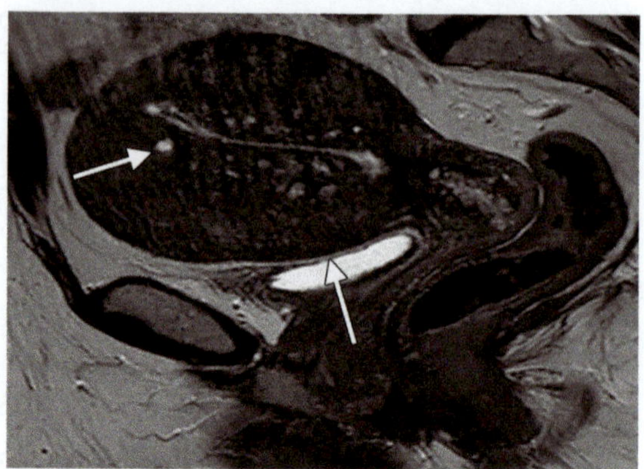

**Fig. 2:** Junctional zone (arrows).

## Junctional Zone

It is consisting of innermost myometrial layer, subvascular layer above the endometrial cavity called archimyometrium and basal endometrial layer. The normal thickness is 7–8 mm as shown in **Figure 2**.

In uterine adenomyosis, it makes the JZ thicker and hazy:

- A JZ of <8 mm is considered unlikely to represent adenomyosis
- A JZ of >12 mm very likely represents adenomyosis.

Once adenomyosis is established, it is thought to progress by epithelial–mesenchymal transition,[3] a process by which epithelial cells become highly motile mesenchymal cells that are capable of migration and invasion, due to loss of cell–cell adhesion properties.

## TYPES OF ADENOMYOSIS

As shown in **Figure 3**, there are three different classification of adenomyosis:

1. *Focal*: It is usually in one particular site of uterus.
2. *Adenomyoma*: It is a form of focal adenomyosis, but it is more extensive, as it results in a uterine mass or benign tumor, similar to uterine fibroma.
3. *Diffuse*: Unlike the other two types, diffuse is spread throughout the uterus.

## IMPACT OF ADENOMYOSIS ON FERTILITY

Adenomyosis may contribute to infertility in many different ways.

### Abnormal Uterotubal Transport

*Anatomical Distortion*

Adenomyoma that distorts the uterine cavity may obstruct the tubal ostia and interfere with sperm migration and embryo transport.

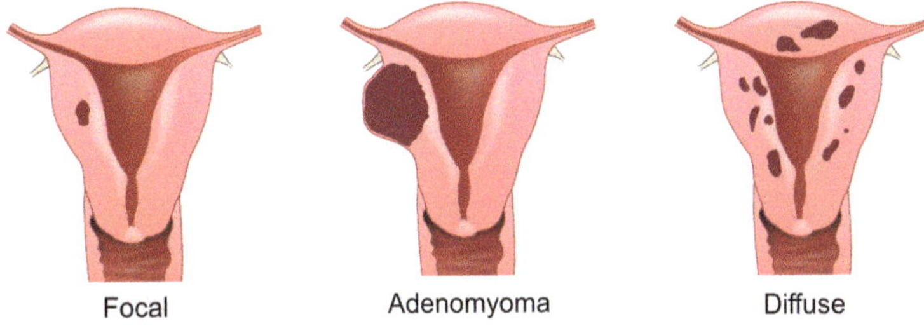



**Fig. 3:** Types of adenomyosis.
*Source:* Seckin Endometriosis Center for Medical Education and Research.

## Problem in Uterine Peristalsis

In women with adenomyosis, normal architecture of the "archimyometrium" (JZ myometrium) was destroyed owing to invagination of the endometrial glands and stroma. This gives dysfunctional uterine hyperperistalsis with increased intrauterine pressure that may affect fertility in patients with adenomyosis.

## Destruction of Myometrial Architecture and Function

Myocytes of adenomyosis are ultrastructurally abnormal and may cause a disturbance in normal calcium cycling in affected myocytes, with subsequent loss of normal rhythmic contraction, eventually affecting uterotubal transport.

## Altered Endometrial Function and Receptivity

### Altered Endometrial Steroid Metabolism

P450arom is an enzyme which is elevated in adenomyosis and it catalyzes the conversion of androgens to estrogens. Clinical pregnancy rates were statistically lower in women with high endometrial P450arom messenger ribonucleic acid (mRNA) levels and they suggest that P450arom mRNA expression can identify women at increased risk of in vitro fertilization (IVF) failure.

### Abnormal Inflammatory Response

Interleukin-1 (IL-1), tumor necrosis factor (TNF), and IL-6 mRNA expression was increased in macrophage-cocultured endometriotic stromal cells in adenomyosis suggesting that an abnormal inflammatory response may impair fertility, refer **Figure 4** below.

### Altered Expression of Estrogen and Progesterone Receptors

Overexpression of estrogen receptor-$\alpha$ (ER-$\alpha$) reduces integrin $\beta$3 secretion in adenomyosis that alters uterine receptivity.

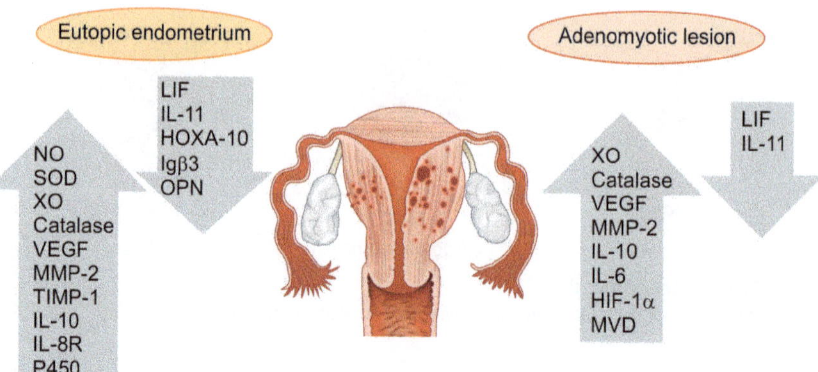


**Fig. 4:** Implantation factors showing altered concentration in adenomyosis-associated infertility. (HIF-1α: hypoxia-inducible factor-1α; Igβ3: immunoglobulin β3; IL-10: interleukin-10; LIF: leukemia inhibitory factor; MMP-2: matrix metalloproteinase-2; MVD: microvascular density; NO: nitric oxide; OPN: osteopontin; SOD: superoxide dismutase; TIMP-1: tissue inhibitor of metalloproteinase-1; VEGF: vascular endothelial growth factor)

## Uterine Oxidative Stress Environmental Dysregulation

Oxidative stress levels do not fluctuate during the menstrual cycle and are overexpressed in adenomyosis and seem to cause infertility.

## Impaired Implantation

### Lack of Expression of Adhesion Molecules

Dysregulation of both integrin β3 and osteopontin (OPN) mRNA and protein in the endometrium during the implantation window suggests that adenomyosis is associated with impaired implantation.

### Reduced Expression of Implantation Markers

Adenomyotic endometrium shows abnormalities in the production of leukemia inhibitory factor (LIF), which may contribute to altering uterine receptivity.

### Altered Function of the Gene for Embryonic Development

*HOXA10* gene, essential for embryonic uterine development and proper adult endometrial growth during the menstrual cycle, may be involved in creating an impairment of implantation in women with adenomyosis.

## ADENOMYOSIS VERSUS ENDOMETRIOSIS

Adenomyosis is similar to endometriosis in some ways, but adenomyosis has different causes and behaves differently.[4] As with endometriosis, adenomyosis occurs when endometrial tissue grows abnormally. With endometriosis, endometrial-like tissue grows outside of the uterus (typically on the fallopian tubes, ovaries, and/or outer surface of the uterus) whereas with adenomyosis, endometrial tissue grows abnormally into the muscle wall of the uterus (called the myometrium). In one study of patients with endometriosis, 78% of women also had adenomyosis.[5]

## STAGING OF ADENOMYOSIS

### Stage 0

Solitary JZ hyperplasia without infiltration of myometrium.

### Stage 1

- *a:* Focal thickening of JZ < 20 mm
- *b:* Focal thickening of JZ > 20 mm.

### Stage 2

- *a:* Diffuse adenomyosis with less than one-third of myometrium involved
- *b:* Diffuse adenomyosis with more than one-third of myometrium involved.

### Stage 3

Uterine adenomyosis and extrauterine localization (RV, bladder).

## DIAGNOSIS

*Meticulous history, examination, and investigation will help to reach the diagnosis.*[6]

### History

It is important to take meticulous history of present and past problems and medical and surgical history.

### Symptoms and Signs

Adenomyosis can vary widely in the type and severity of symptoms that it causes, ranging from being entirely asymptomatic 33% of the time to being a severe and debilitating condition in some cases. Women with adenomyosis typically first report symptoms when they are between 40 and 50 years, but symptoms can occur in younger women.

Symptoms and the estimated percent affected may include:

- Chronic pelvic pain (70–77%)[7]
- *Menstrual problems:*
  - Prolonged menstrual cramping or dysmenorrhea (15–30%)
  - Heavy menstrual bleeding (40–60%), which is more common within women with deeper adenomyosis

- • Longer than normal menstrual cycles
- • Clots during menstrual bleeding can also be a symptom of adenomyosis
- • Spotting between menstrual cycles
- Painful sexual intercourse (7–8%)
- Infertility or subfertility (11–12%)
- A bearing down feeling and dragging sensation down thighs and legs
- Painful bowel movement (dyschezia)
- Bladder symptoms including—pressure on bladder, uncomfortable urination (dysuria), burning urination, or blood in the urine (hematuria)
- Peripheral nerve numbness or weakness (neuropathy), which can cause leg or bowel pain during periods.

*Clinical signs of adenomyosis may include*:

- *Uterine enlargement (30%)*:
  - • Bulky, boggy, and globular enlargement, which, in turn, can lead to symptoms of pelvic fullness as shown in **Figure 5**.
  - • Tender uterus
  - • Sometimes, if associated with endometriosis, it will be fixed and retroverted.

*Women with adenomyosis are also more likely to have other uterine conditions*:

- Uterine fibroids (35–50%)
- Endometriosis (40–51%)
- Endometrial polyp (3–7%)
- Atypical endometrial hyperplasia (3–3.5%)
- Adenocarcinoma (1.4%).

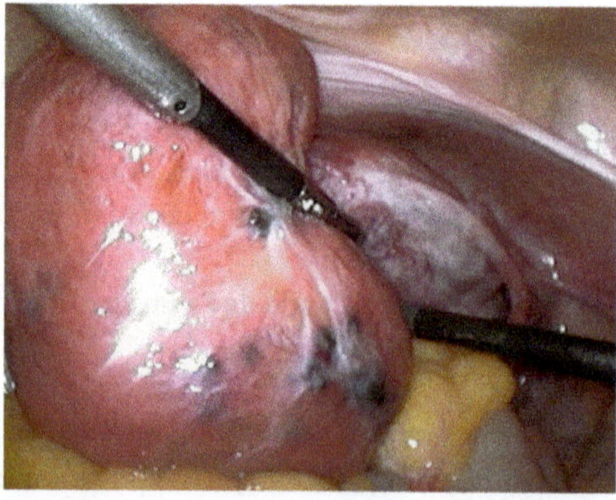

**Fig. 5:** Laparoscopic view of boggy uterine enlargement in adenomyosis.

## Impact on Pregnancy Outcome

If a patient with adenomyosis is pregnant, it may cause adverse pregnancy outcomes:

- Increased risk of second-trimester miscarriage
- Pregnancy-induced hypertension
- Preeclampsia
- Abnormal placentation
- Cervical incompetency
- Preterm premature rupture of membranes
- Preterm birth (PTB)
- Small for gestational age (SGA) fetuses
- Fetal malpresentation
- Increased incidence of cesarean delivery
- Postpartum hemorrhage.

## Imaging

*Advancement of imaging technique has significantly helps the diagnosis.*

Transvaginal sonography (TVS) and magnetic resonance imaging (MRI) can both be used to strongly suggest the diagnosis of adenomyosis, guide treatment options, and monitor response to treatment. Indeed, transvaginal ultrasonography (TVUS) and MRI are the only two practical means available to establish a presurgical diagnosis. TVS is often preferred because it is more widely available and significantly more cost-effective for the patients.[8]

### Transvaginal Sonography

Transvaginal ultrasonography has a sensitivity of 79–90% and a specificity of 85-93% for the detection of adenomyosis.[9] **Figure 6** shows how adenomyosis appears under TVS.

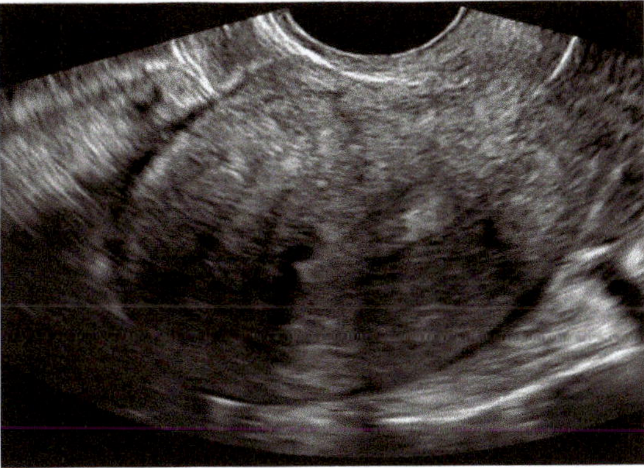

**Fig. 6:** Transvaginal sonographic findings of adenomyosis.

It may be useful to categorize ultrasound findings into three groups that mirror the histological findings:

1. *Adeno—Ectopic endometrial glands*:
   - Subendometrial echogenic linear striations and/or nodules (specific sign), extending from endometrium and into inner myometrium
   - Hyperechoic islands
   - Irregular endometrial-myometrial junction
   - Tiny (1–5 mm) anechoic myometrial and subendometrial cysts (specific sign): Reflecting glands filled with fluid
   - Cystic striations.

2. *Myosis—Muscular hyperplasia ± Hypertrophy, which may be hypoechoic*:
   - Focal or diffuse myometrial bulkiness, which may be asymmetric:
     - Typically of the fundal region and posterior wall
   - Focal lesions have relatively indistinct borders, compared to leiomyomas
   - Asymmetrical myometrial thickening
   - Thickening of the transition zone can sometimes be visualized as a hypoechoic halo surrounding the endometrial layer of ≥12 mm thickness (less specific).

3. *Vascularity—Flow on color Doppler*:
   - Generally increased
   - Increased number of tortuous vessels penetrating myometrium
   - Areas of increased vascularity reciprocate distribution of lesions.

A *Venetian blind or rain shower appearance* (linear striations, parallel shadowing) may be seen as a combination of *heterogeneous* is not dissimilar to the appearance of chronic liver parenchymal disease—hence *cirrhosis of the uterus*.[10]

*Doppler ultrasonography* can be used to differentiate adenomyomas from uterine fibroids as shown in **Figure 7**. This is because uterine fibroids typically

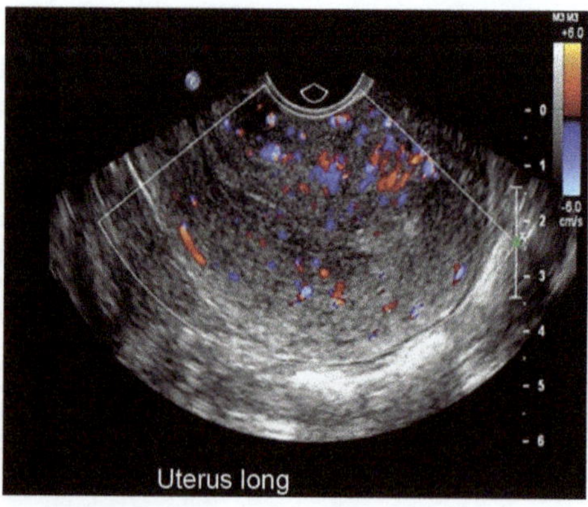


**Fig. 7:** Transvaginal color Doppler findings of adenomyosis.

have blood vessels circling the fibroids capsule. In contrast, adenomyomas are characterized by widespread blood vessels within the lesion. Doppler ultrasonography also serves to differentiate the static fluid within myometrial cysts from flowing blood within vessels.[11-13]

## MRI

Pelvic MRI is the modality of choice to diagnose and characterize adenomyosis. Small field of view T2-weighted images (sagittal and axial) are most useful.[14,15] MRI has a sensitivity of 78–88% and a specificity of 67–93%.

The most easily recognized feature is thickening of the JZ ≥ 12 mm, either diffusely or focally (normal JZ thickness is up to ~5 mm):

- *T1*:
  - Foci of high T1 signal are often seen, indicating menstrual hemorrhage into the ectopic endometrial tissues.[16]
- *T2*:
  - Typically, a region of adenomyosis appears as an ill-defined ovoid/ diffuse region of thickening, often with small high T2 signal regions representing small areas of cystic change
  - The region may also have a striated appearance.
- *T1 contrast + Gadolinium*:
  - Contrast-enhanced MRI evaluation is usually not required for evaluation of adenomyosis; however, if performed, it shows enhancement of the ectopic endometrial glands.[17]

Interspersed within the thickened, darker signal of the JZ, one will often see foci of hyperintensity (bright spots) on the T2-weighted scans representing small cystically dilatated glands or more acute sites of microhemorrhage.[18]

MRI is limited by other factors, but not by calcified uterine fibroids (as in ultrasound). In particular, MRI is better able to differentiate adenomyosis from multiple small uterine fibroids as shown in **Figures 8 to 11**.

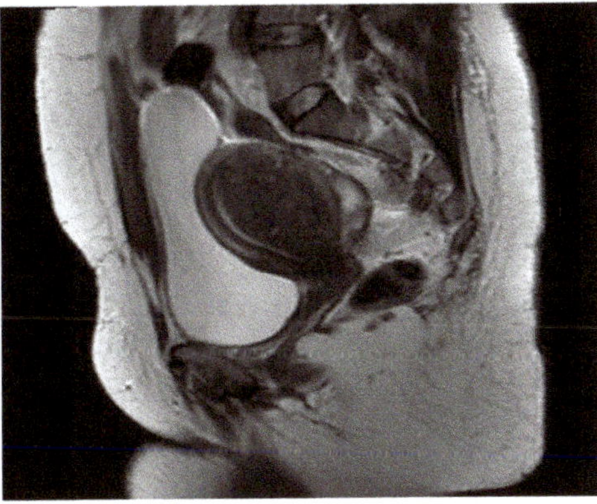

**Fig. 8:** Focal adenomyosis.

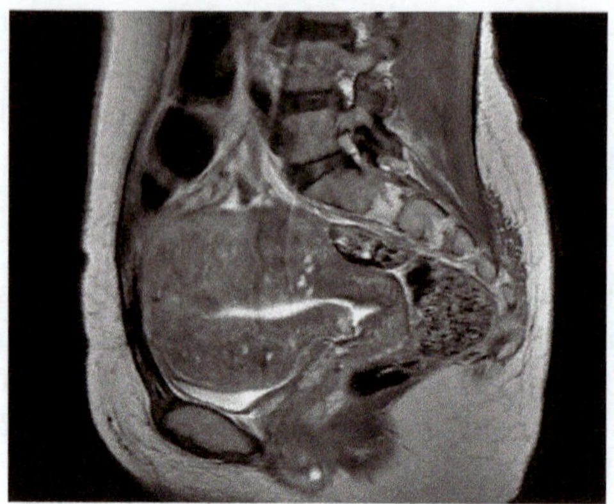

**Fig. 9:** Diffuse adenomyosis.

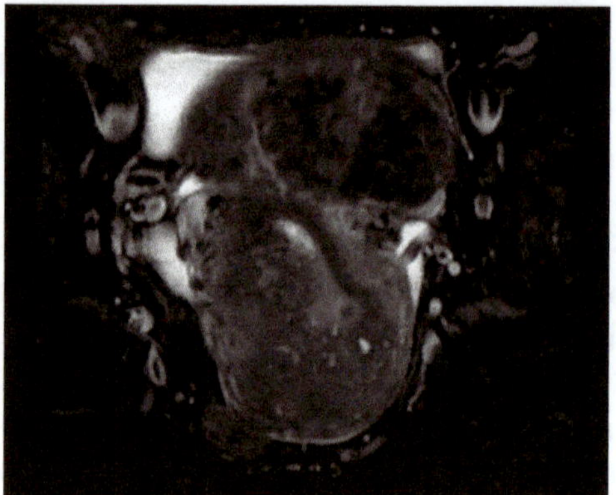

**Fig. 10:** Adenomyosis with concurrent fibroid.

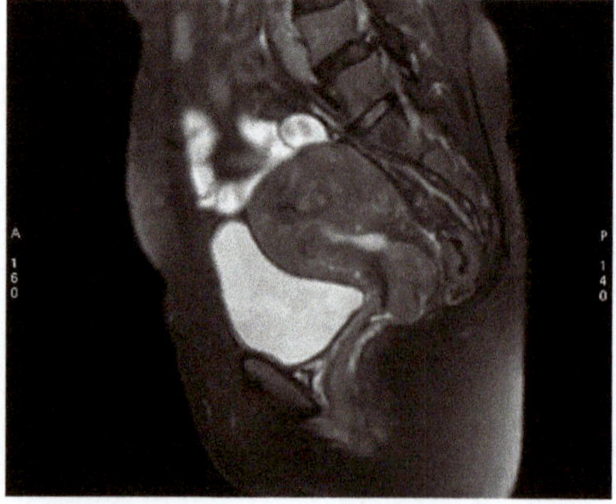

**Fig. 11:** Adenomyosis with concurrent polyp.

## Hysterosalpingogram

As shown in **Figure 12**, adenomyosis diverticula extending into the myometrium under HSG view.

## CT Scan

- CT is insensitive for adenomyosis, but may demonstrate resulting uterine enlargement as shown in **Figure 13**.
- Distinguishing adenomyosis and uterine fibroids on CT are challenging, although the presence of calcifications strongly favor it.[19]

## Hysteroscopy

Diagnostic hysteroscopy does not provide pathognomonic signs for adenomyosis, although the presence of an irregular endometrium with endometrial defects, altered vascularization, and cystic hemorrhagic lesions can be possibly associated with the entity.[20] In addition to the

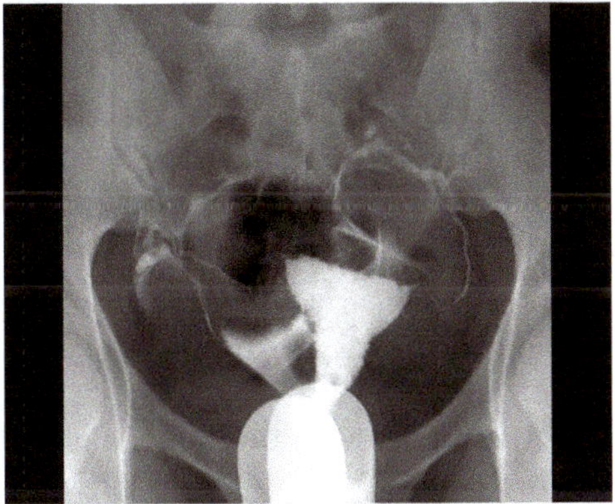

**Fig. 12:** Hysterosalpingogram (HSG) finding of adenomyosis.

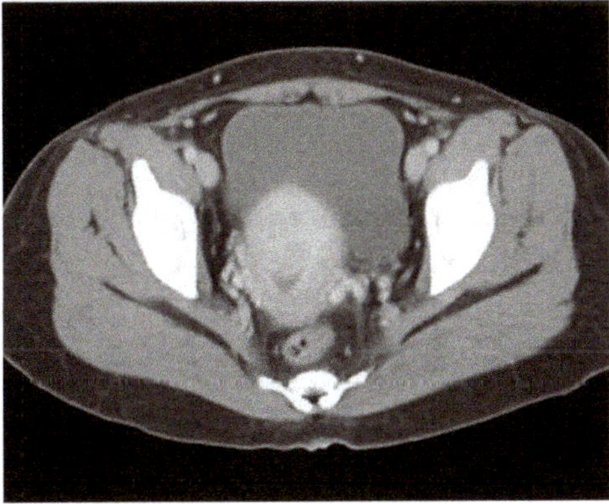

**Fig. 13:** CT scan of adenomyosis.

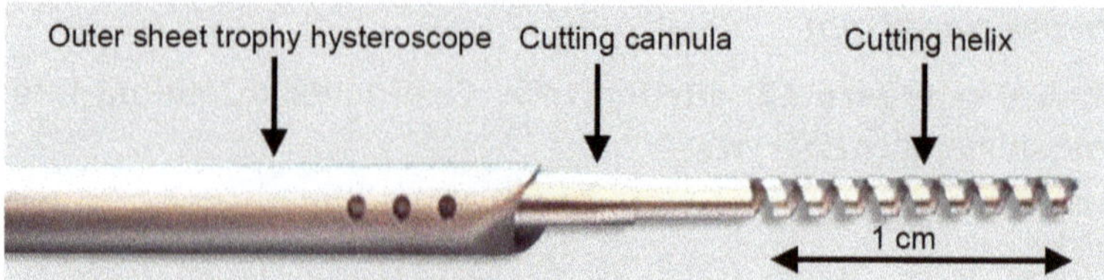


**Fig. 14:** Hysteroscope showing outer 7 inner cannulas.

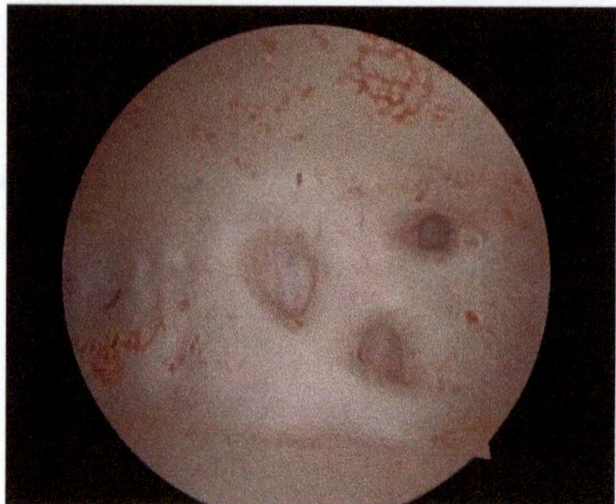

**Fig. 15:** Hysteroscopy image of adenomyosis. Small openings at the endometrial surface can be seen during hysteroscopy.

direct visualization of the uterine cavity, the hysteroscopic approach offers the possibility of obtaining endometrial/myometrial biopsies under visual control.

The utero-spirotome operates with two devices in tandem: (1) the receiving needle with a cutting helix at the distal end and (2) a cutting cannula as an outer sheet as shown in **Figure 14**. The correct direction and position of the helix point is under continuous ultrasonographic imaging and hysteroscopic control.[21] Under ultrasound guidance, the spirotome can be directed toward any intramural localized lesion such as cystic adenomyosis, thus creating a visible hysteroscopic channel that allows access to the cystic cavity.

*Natural access to junctional zone myometrium by hysteroscopy:*
- Subtle lesions sign of JZ pathology
- Abnormal endometrial images **(Fig. 15)** with an unclear clinical significance
- Strawberry pattern
- Cystic mucosal elevation
- Focal or general hypervascularization
- Endometrial defects.

Sometimes, it is suggested that the combination of TVS, fluid hysteroscopy, and contrast sonography can be a powerful tool for detecting endometrial and myometrial abnormalities in association with adenomyosis.[22]

## TREATMENT

- *Home remedies to treat adenomyosis*: Sometimes, some home remedies help to get rid from symptoms of adenomyosis such as heating pads, massage with essential oils, castor oil, Shepherd's purse, ginger, turmeric, calcium, magnesium, aloe vera, vitamins, apple, cider, and vinegar.[23]
- *Medical*: Medical treatment for adenomyosis is similar to those given for endometriosis. Apart from symptomatic relief, hormonal treatment mainly works by inhibition of ovulation, cessation of menses, improving the hormonal milieu, and causing decidualization of the endometrial deposits:
    - *Nonsteroidal anti-inflammatory drugs (NSAIDs)*: They will work by inhibiting the cyclooxygenase (COX-1 and COX-2) and decreasing the production of prostaglandins. NSAIDs have been proved to be effective in the treatment of primary dysmenorrhea.
    - *Oral contraceptive pills (OCPs)*: Combined OCPs work by inhibiting ovulation by suppressing the release of gonadotropins. Many studies have shown that they are effective in the treatment of dysmenorrhea. A prospective observational trial showed that continuous low-dose OCP was more effective than cyclical low-dose OCP in controlling symptoms in patients after surgical treatment for adenomyosis.[24]
    - *Danazol*: Danazol is an isoxazol derivative of 12-alpha-ethinyltesto-sterone. It causes a hypogonadic state and thus is widely used for the treatment of AUB in adenomyosis. However, data on its use in adenomyosis remains limited. This may be due to its unwanted adverse effects after systemic treatment device in 14 women. During insertion of the danazol-loaded intrauterine device (IUD), there was complete remission of dysmenorrhea in some patients.
    - *Dienogest*: Dienogest is a selective synthetic oral progestin that combines the pharmacological properties of 17-alpha-progesterone and 19-norprogesterone with pronounced local effect on endometrial tissue. Dienogest has been shown to be effective in the treatment of endometriosis-associated pelvic pain. A prospective clinical trial has shown dienogest to be a valuable alternative to depot triptorelin acetate for treatment of premenopausal pelvic pains in women with uterine adenomyosis.[25]
    - *Levonorgestrel-releasing intrauterine device (LNG-IUD)*: LNG-IUD is an intrauterine device, which release 20 µg of levonorgestrel per day. It has been shown to be an effective treatment for AUB.

LNG-IUD acts locally and causes decidualization of the endometrium and adenomyotic deposits. LNG-IUD alleviates dysmenorrhea by improving uterine contractility and reducing local prostaglandin production within the endometrium. LNG-IUD appears to be an effective method in relieving dysmenorrhea associated with adenomyosis and more effective than the combined OCP, improved the quality-of-life, and appears to be a promising alternative treatment to hysterectomy:

- Levonorgestrel-releasing intrauterine device may be used in conjunction with other treatment modalities such as gonadotropin-releasing hormone (GnRH) analog or transcervical resection of the endometrium (TCRE). In the latter study, it was found that TCRE combined with LNG-IUD was more effective in reducing menstrual flow compared with the LNG-IUD alone, although there was no significant difference in the amount of pain reduction between the two treatment strategies.[26]

- *Gonadotropin-releasing hormone agonists*: GnRH agonists are effective in alleviating dysmenorrhea and relieving menorrhagia associated with adenomyosis. However, due to the undesirable climacteric side effects and risk of osteoporosis, treatment with GnRH agonists is usually restricted to a short duration of 3–6 months, although the duration of use may be extended if add-back estrogen therapy is employed. Discontinuation of treatment usually leads to regrowth of the lesions and recurrence of symptoms.

- *Selective estrogen receptor modulators (SERMs)*: SERMs such as tamoxifen or raloxifene have been tried in the treatment of endometriosis based on observations that SERMs may reduce endometriosis lesion in mouse; however, their value in the treatment of adenomyoma has not been formally explored.[27]

- *Aromatase inhibitors*: Adenomyotic deposits are estrogen dependent. Aromatase inhibitors inhibit the conversion of estrogen from androgens, thereby lowering the synthesis of estrogen. A prospective randomized controlled study found that the efficacy of aromatase inhibitors (letrozole 2.5 mg/day) in reducing the volume of adenomyoma as well as improving adenomyosis symptoms was similar to that of GnRH agonists (goserelin 3.6 mg/month).

- *Ulipristal acetate (UPA)*: It is a potent selective progesterone receptor modulator. There is good evidence to suggest that it can be used to shrink fibroid and control menorrhagia. It is possible that it may be similarly effective in the treatment of adenomyoma, but literature data is lacking.

- *Antiplatelet therapy*: There is new evidence to suggest a role of antiplatelet therapy in treating adenomyosis. Emerging evidence suggests that endometriotic lesions are wounds undergoing repeated tissue injury and repair (ReTIAR) and platelets induce epithelial–mesenchymal transition (EMT) and fibroblast-to-myofibroblast transdifferentiation (FMT), leading ultimately to fibrosis. Adenomyotic lesions are thought to have similar pathogenesis to that of endometriosis. A recent study in mice suggests that antiplatelet treatment may suppress myometrial infiltration, improve generalized hyperalgesia, and reduce uterine hyperactivity.

## Surgery

The objective of surgical management is to ameliorate symptoms in a conservative manner, by excision or cytoreduction of adenomyotic lesions, while preserving, even improving, fertility.[28-30] The choice of procedure depends, ultimately, on the location and extent of disease, the patient's desire for uterine preservation and fertility, and surgical skill.[28]

Historically, hysterectomy was used to treat adenomyosis; for patients declining fertility preservation, hysterectomy remains the definitive treatment. Since the early 1950s, several techniques for laparotomic reduction have been developed. Surgeries that achieve partial reduction include:

- *Uterine-sparing procedures*:
  - *Wedge resection of the uterine wall* entails removal of the seromuscular layer at the identified location of adenomyotic tissue, with subsequent repair of the remaining muscular and serosal layers surrounding the wound. Because adenomyotic tissue can remain on either side of the incision in wedge resection, clinical improvement in symptoms of dysmenorrhea and menorrhagia is modest and recurrence is possible.
  - *Modified reduction surgery*: Modifications of reduction surgery include slicing adenomyotic tissue using microsurgery and partial excision.
  - *Transverse H-incision of the uterine wall* involves a transverse incision on the uterine fundus, separating serosa and myometrium, followed by removal of diseased tissue using an electrosurgical scalpel or scissors. Tensionless suturing is used to close the myometrial layers in one or two layers to establish hemostasis and closes the defect; serosal flaps are closed with subserosal interrupted sutures. Data show that, following surgery with this technique, 21.4–38.7% of patients who attempt conception achieve clinical pregnancy.

    Complete, conservative resection in cases of diffuse and focal adenomyosis is possible using the triple-flap method, in which total resection is achieved by removing diseased myometrium until healthy, soft tissue—with normal texture, color, and vascularity—is reached. Repair with this technique reduces the risk of uterine rupture by reconstructing the uterine wall using a muscle flap prepared by metroplasty.[16] In a study of 64 women who underwent triple-flap resection, a clinical pregnancy rate of 74% and a live birth rate of 52% were reported.

- *Minimally invasive approaches*: Although several techniques have been developed for focal excision of adenomyosis by laparotomy, the trend has been toward minimally invasive surgery, which reduces estimated blood loss, decreases length of stay, and reduces adhesion formation—all without a statistically significant difference in long-term clinical outcomes, compared to other techniques. Furthermore, enhanced visualization of pelvic organs provided by laparoscopy is vital in the case of adenomyosis.

- *Endomyometrial ablation or resection*: There is limited report on the use of laparoscopic or hysteroscopic endometrial in treating adenomyosis in the literature. The success rate of myometrial electrocoagulation ranges from 55 to 70% as reported.

- *Uterine artery embolization (UAE)*: As shown in **Figure 16**, this is minimally invasive procedure, doctors intentionally block two large arteries that supply the uterus, called the uterine arteries. This

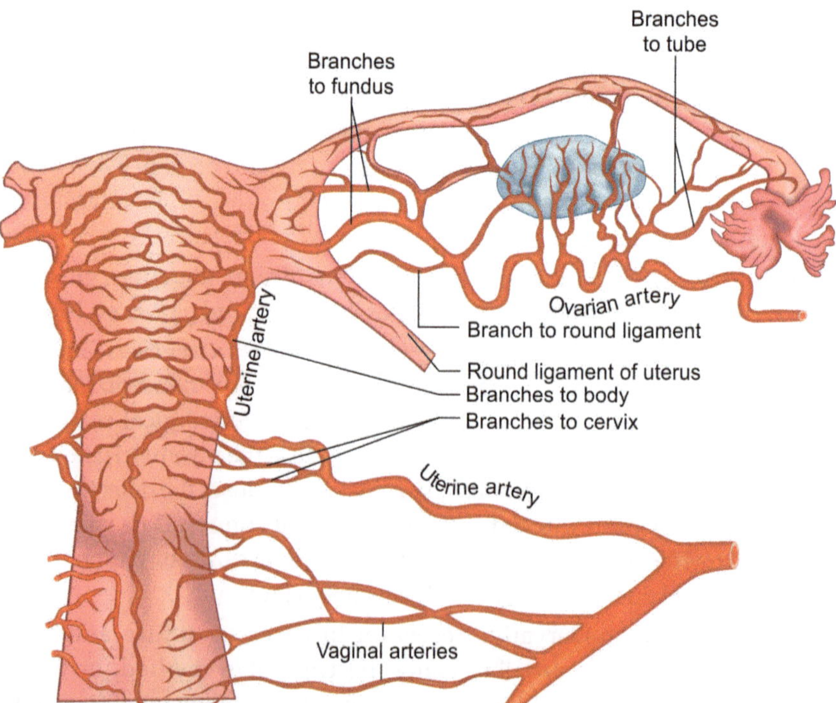


**Fig. 16:** Uterine artery embolization.

is performed in order to dramatically reduce the blood supply to the uterus. By doing so, there is insufficient blood and thus oxygen present for the adenomyosis to develop and spread. 57–75% of women who undergo UAE for adenomyosis typically report long-term improvement in their menstrual pain and bleeding. However, there is a recurrence rate of symptoms in 35% of women following a UAE. Also, UAE has the risk of causing major complications in 5% of women who undergo the procedure. Major complications include infection, significant bleeding, and needing an additional surgery. UAE has also been shown in some cases to reduce ovarian function. Finally, 26% of women who undergo UAE ultimately end up requiring a hysterectomy.

- *High-intensity focused ultrasound (HIFU)*: HIFU is another nonsurgical treatment for uterine fibroids that focuses high-intensity ultrasound in the target lesion causing coagulative necrosis and shrinkage of the lesion. Both MRI and USG can be used for guidance for the procedure. MRI has better real-time thermal mapping during the HIFU treatment. Yet, ultrasound-guided HIFU is less costly and offers real-time anatomic monitoring imaging and a grayscale change during treatment represents a reliable indicator in treatment response. It is effective in both focal and diffuse lesions.

■ *Nonuterine-sparing procedures*:

- *Hysterectomy*: Surgical removal of the uterus has historically been the primary method of diagnosing and treating adenomyosis. It was especially popular in women who had completed their childbearing or in cases where fertility was not desired. Today, there are many more medical and surgical interventions available. These treatments, such as hormonal therapy and endometrial ablation, have significantly reduced the number of women who require a hysterectomy. That being said, hysterectomies remain as the final treatment option for women in whom the other treatments have failed. Typically viewed as definitive treatment for the bleeding and pelvic pain associated with adenomyosis, hysterectomy will always result in sterility and cessation of menstrual bleeding. Pelvic pain, on the other hand, can persist after a hysterectomy in as many as 22% of women.

## Treatment Options for Fertility Restoration

Previously, when adenomyosis was diagnosed in fourth or fifth decade of parous women with history of menorrhagia and dysmenorrhea—hysterectomy was the treatment of choice. Even now in young women when the size of uterus exceeds 10 cm (>12 weeks gravid uterus size)—presenting with menorrhagia and dysmenorrhea—hysterectomy with preservation of ovaries for future surrogacy is still considered to be the rational treatment. But nowadays, there are varieties of fertility preservation management.

They are: GnRH analog, conservative surgery with GnRH, LNG containing IUS, high-intensity focused USG, UAE, and laparoscopic partial resection of uterus with uterine artery occlusion.

## IMPACT OF ADENOMYOSIS ON ASSISTED REPRODUCTIVE TECHNOLOGY

Adenomyosis usually has negative impact on pregnancy outcome due to prolonged downregulation with difficulty of ovarian stimulation for IVF. In addition, bad quality of oocyte and implantation failures are the others factors of poor outcome of assisted reproductive technology (ART).

## HISTOLOGY

On gross inspection, the uterus with diffuse adenomyosis is uniformly enlarged and boggy, in contrast to the irregular and firm appearance of the fibroid uterus, although the two conditions (fibroids and adenomyosis) can occur concurrently. The average uterine weight is usually between 80 and 200 g, unless coexisting leiomyomas are present. Upon sectioning the uterus, the myometrial wall appears thickened and often contains small hemorrhagic or chocolate-colored areas representing islands of endometrial bleeding **(Fig. 17)**. Adenomyosis can be present diffusely throughout the myometrium or confined to a discrete area (termed an adenomyoma). Adenomyomas can clinically resemble leiomyomas.

The term "cystic" is used to describe either diffuse adenomyosis or adenomyomas for which cysts ≥1 cm in diameter are seen on imaging studies. The entity "juvenile cystic adenomyoma" has been used, mainly in reports

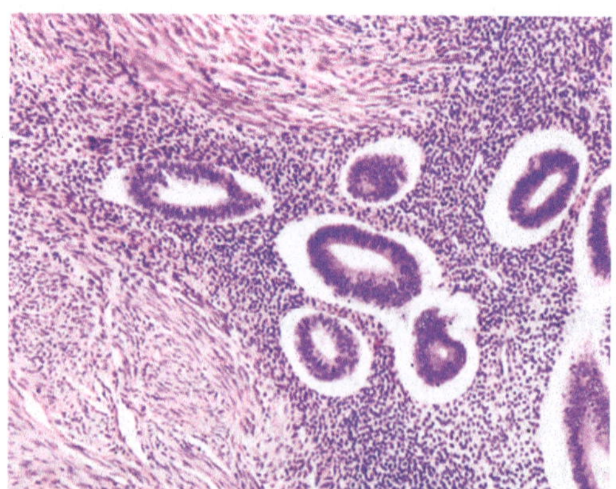

**Fig. 17:** Histopathologic image of adenomyosis showing nonfunctioning hyperplasia-like endometrial island.

from Japan, to describe a syndrome in which women 30 years or younger with severe dysmenorrhea have myometrial cysts ≥1 cm.[31] However, authors from other countries have reported cystic adenomyosis in women of a variety of reproductive ages.[3]

The pathognomonic feature of adenomyosis is the presence of endometrial tissue within the myometrium at a distance of at least one low power field (some authorities insist on two low power fields) from the endomyometrial junction. The distance requirement is to preclude mistaking the normal endometrium between muscle fibers at the mucosa for adenomyosis when the specimen is transected for slide preparation. The widespread use of endometrial ablation potentially could confound the diagnosis as the procedure distorts or destroys the endometrial–myometrial junction.

## PROGNOSIS

Adenomyosis is a benign but often progressing condition. It is advocated that adenomyosis poses no increased risk for cancer development. However, both entities could coexist and the endometrial tissue within the myometrium could harbor endometrioid adenocarcinoma, with potentially deep myometrial invasion. As the condition is estrogen dependent, menopause presents a natural cure. Ultrasound features of adenomyosis will still be present after menopause. People with adenomyosis are also more likely to have uterine fibroids or endometriosis.

## PATIENT EDUCATION

It is important to proper counsel the patients about the disease, diagnostic approaches, laboratory investigation, and exclude others differential diagnosis. When adenomyosis is suspected or diagnosis is made, we need to discuss the pathophysiology and natural history of the disease with the patient. It is a time demanding approach to discuss the patient about the options of treatment and recent modern techniques of management.

## PREVENTION

As the exact cause of adenomyosis is unknown, it is recommended that every woman have an annual physical examination, pelvic examination, and cervical cancer screening in order to detect the early abnormality.

## LONG-TERM OUTLOOK

Adenomyosis is not life-threatening. Many treatments are available to help alleviate your symptoms. A hysterectomy is the only treatment that can eliminate them altogether. However, the condition often goes away on its own after menopause.

Adenomyosis is not the same as endometriosis. This condition occurs when the endometrial tissues become implanted outside of the uterus. Women with adenomyosis may also have or develop endometriosis.

## CONCLUSION

Many treatment modalities are now available for the treatment of adenomyosis. The management plan ought to be individualized, depending on the presenting symptom and the desire to achieve a successful pregnancy. Recent development in various nonsurgical and surgical options has significantly improved the prospect of a successful treatment in women wishing to conceive again.

## KEY PRACTICE POINTS

- Adenomyosis is common and benign, but remains underdiagnosed because of a nonspecific clinical presentation and lack of standardized diagnostic criteria
- Adenomyosis can cause significant associated morbidity: dysmenorrhea, HMB, chronic pelvic pain, and infertility
- High clinical suspicion warrants evaluation by imaging
- Medical management is largely aimed at ameliorating symptoms
- Impact on fertility is significant and ART outcome is poor
- A patient who does not respond to medical treatment or does not desire pregnancy has a variety of surgical options; the extent of disease and the patient's wish for uterine preservation guide the selection of surgical technique
- Hysterectomy is the definitive treatment but, in patients who want to avoid radical resection, techniques developed for laparotomy are available, to allow conservative resection using laparoscopy
- Ideally, surgery is performed using a combined laparoscopy and minila- parotomy approach, after appropriate imaging.

## REFERENCES


1. Pearce CL, Templeman C, Rossing MA, Lee A, Near AM, Webb PM, et al. Association between endometriosis and risk of histological subtypes of ovarian cancer: a pooled analysis of case-control studies. Lancet Oncol. 2012;13(4):385-94.
2. Kitawaki J. Adenomyosis: the pathophysiology of an oestrogen-dependent disease. Best Pract Res Clin Obstet Gynaecol. 2006;20(4):493-502.
3. Cheong Y, Stones W. Investigations for chronic pelvic pain. Revs Gynaecol Pract. 2005;5(4):227-36.
4. Olive DL, Schwartz LB. Endometriosis. N Engl J Med. 1993;328(24):1759-69.
5. Templeman C, Marshall SF, Ursin G, Horn-Ross PL, Clarke CA, Allen M, et al. Adenomyosis and endometriosis in the California Teachers Study. Fertil Steril. 2008;90(2):415-24.

6. Kok VC, Tsai HJ, Su CF, Lee CK. The risks for ovarian, endometrial, breast, colorectal, and other cancers in women with newly diagnosed endometriosis or adenomyosis: a population-based study. Int J Gynecol Cancer: official journal of the International Gynecological Cancer Society. 2015;25(6):968-76.

7. Kvaskoff M, Mu F, Terry KL, Harris HR, Poole EM, Farland L, et al. Endometriosis: a high-risk population for major chronic diseases? Hum Reprod Update. 2015;21(4):500-16.

8. Gun I, Oner O, Bodur S, Ozdamar O, Atay V. Is adenomyosis associated with the risk of endometrial cancer? Medicinski Glasnik: official publication of the Medical Association of Zenica-Doboj Canton, Bosnia and Herzegovina. 2012;9(2):268-72.

9. Matsuo K, Cahoon SS, Gualtieri M, Scannell CA, Jung CE, Takano T, et al. Significance of adenomyosis on tumor progression and survival outcome of endometrial cancer. Ann Surg Oncol. 2014;21(13):4246-55.

10. Taneichi A, Fujiwara H, Takahashi Y, Takei Y, Machida S, Saga Y, et al. Influences of uterine adenomyosis on muscle invasion and prognosis of endometrioid adenocarcinoma. Int J Gynecol Cancer: official journal of the International Gynecological Cancer Society. 2014;24(8):1429-33.

11. Leyendecker G, Bilgicyildirim A, Inacker M, et al. Adenomyosis and endometriosis. Re-visiting their association and further insights into the mechanisms of autotraumatization. An MRI study. Arch Gynecol Obstet. 2015;291(4):917-7.

12. Vannuccini S, Luisi S, Tosti C, et al. Role of medical therapy in the management of uterine adenomyosis. Fertil Steril. 2018;109(3):398-405.

13. Carrarelli P, Yen CF, Arcuri F, et al. Myostatin, follistatin and activin type II receptors are highly expressed in adenomyosis. Fertil Steril. 2015;104(3):744-52.e1

14. Carrarelli P, Yen CF, Funghi L, et al. Expression of inflammatory and neurogenic mediators in adenomyosis. Reprod Sci. 2016;24(3):369 75.

15. García-Solares J, Donnez J, Donnez O, et al. Pathogenesis of uterine adenomyosis: invagination or metaplasia? Fertil Steril. 2018;109(3):371-9.

16. Koike N, Tsunemi T, Uekuri C, Akasaka J, Ito F, Shigemitsu A, et al. Pathogenesis and malignant transformation of adenomyosis (review). Oncol Rep. 2013;29(3):861-7.

17. Brosens I, Derwig I, Brosens J, et al. The enigmatic uterine junctional zone: the missing link between reproductive disorders and major obstetrical disorders? Hum Reprod. 2010;25(3):569-74.

18. Benagiano G, Brosens I, Habiba M. Structural and molecular features of the endomyometrium in endometriosis and adenomyosis. Hum Reprod Update. 2014;20(3):386-402.

19. Shaked S, Jaffa AJ, Grisaru D, et al. Uterine peristalsis-induced stresses within the uterine wall may sprout adenomyosis. Biomech Model Mechanobiol. 2015;14(3):437-44.

20. Gargett CE, Schwab KE, Deane JA. Endometrial stem/progenitor cells: the first 10 years. Hum Reprod Update. 2016;22(2):137-63.

21. Chan RW, Schwab KE, Gargett CE. Clonogenicity of human endometrial epithelial and stromal cells. Biol Reprod. 2004;70(6):1738-50.

22. Chapron C, Tosti C, Marcellin L, et al. Relationship between the magnetic resonance imaging appearance of adenomyosis and endometriosis phenotypes. Hum Reprod. 2017;32(7):1393-401.

23. Marcellin L, Santulli P, Bortolato S, et al. Anterior focal adenomyosis and bladder deep infiltrating endometriosis: is there a link? J Minim Invasive Gynecol. 2018;25(5):896-901.

24. Kim MD, Kim NK, Kim HJ, Lee MH. Pregnancy following uterine artery embolization with polyvinyl alcohol particles for patients with uterine fibroid or adenomyosis. Cardiovasc Intervent Radiol. 2005;28:611-5.

25. Kitamura Y, Allison SJ, Jha RC, Spies JB, Flick PA, Ascher SM. MRI of adenomyosis: changes with uterine artery embolization. Am J Roentgenol. 2006;186(3):855-64.

26. Furman B, Appelman Z, Hagay Z, Caspi B. Alcohol sclerotherapy for successful treatment of focal adenomyosis: a case report. Ultrasound Obstet Gynecol. 2007;29(4): 460-2.

27. Yang Z, Cao YD, Hu LN, Wang ZB. Feasibility of laparoscopic high-intensity focused ultrasound treatment for patients with uterine localized adenomyosis. Fertil Steril. 2009 ;91(6):2338-43.

28. Kroon N, Reginald P. Medical management of chronic pelvic pain. Curr Obs Gynae. 2005;15(5):285-90.

29. Musa F, Frey MK, Im HB, Chekmareva M, Ellenson LH, Holcomb K. Does the presence of adenomyosis and lymphovascular space invasion affect lymph node status in patients with endometrioid adenocarcinoma of the endometrium? Am J Obstet Gynecol. 2012;207(5):417e1-6.

30. Donnez J, Nisolle M. Peritoneal endometriosis, ovarian endometriosis and "endometriotic" nodules of the rectovaginal septum are three different entities. Gynecol Obstet. 1995;3:121-3.

31. Farquhar C, Brosens I. Medical and surgical management of adenomyosis. Best Pract Res Clin Obstet Gynaecol. 2006;20(4):603-16.

# Index

Page numbers followed by *f* refer to figure and *t* refer to table.

## K

Keloid 13

## L

Laparoscopic cyst enucleation 28
Laparoscopic excision 40, 98*f*
Laparoscopic resection 107*f*
Laparoscopic surgery 73*f*
Laparoscopic surgical techniques 109
Laparoscopic uterine nerve ablation 73
Laparoscopic uterosacral nerve ablation 47
Laparoscopy 11, 12, 46, 47, 68, 80, 97
    advantages of 25
    diagnostic 22
Laparotomy 12, 47, 97
Leiomyoma 130
Letrozole 40, 58
    plus triptorelin 40
Leukemia inhibitory factor 136*f*
Leuprolide 38, 56
    acetate 29, 39
    depot 56
Levonorgestrel 37, 38
    releasing intrauterine system 24, 37, 70,
        145, 146
Lipoma 13
Luteal insufficiency 8
Luteal phase defect 95
Luteinized unruptured follicle syndrome 8,
        9, 95
Luteinizing hormone 9, 38, 39, 58, 86, 121
Lymphatic spread, Halban's theory of 101
Lynestrenol 116

## M

Macrophages 95
Magnetic resonance imaging 11, 22, 35, 96,
        96*f*, 106, 139, 141
Malignancy 12, 130
Matrix metalloproteinase 114, 136*f*
Medroxyprogesterone 38
    acetate 57, 71, 116
Megestrol acetate 57
Membranes, preterm premature rupture of
        139
Menarche, early age of 4
Menopause, late 4
Menses, irregular 21
Menstrual cycles 4, 34, 138
Menstrual pain, severe 94
Messenger ribonucleic acid 135
Metaplasia theory 2
Meyer and Ivanoff theory 101
Migraine 21
Minimal endometriosis, typical appearance
    of 1*f*
Minimally invasive approaches 148
Miscarriage, second-trimester 139
Molecular tests 97

Monocyte chemoattractant protein-1 114
Müllerian anomalies 21
Multicentral disease 109
Multifocal disease 109
Muscle 13
Musculoskeletal disorders 21
Myometrial architecture, destruction of 135
Myometrium 137
Myosis 140
Mysterious disease 77

## N

Nafarelin 38, 56
National Institute for Health and Care
        Excellence 24
Nerve
    growth factor 115
    infiltration of 34
    interrupting surgeries 42
    irritation of 34
Neurogenesis 34
Nodular excision 109
Nodules, malignant 13
Noninvasive therapy 61
Nonsteroidal anti-inflammatory drugs 7, 23,
        26, 35, 55, 70, 116, 145
    role of 70
Nonuterine-sparing procedures 149
Norethindrone 37, 38
    acetate 25, 57
Norethisterone 116
    acetate 39
Norgestrel 37
Nuclear factor-kappa b 68

## O

Oocytes, quality of 78
Oophorectomy 42
Operative laparoscopy 51
Oral Chinese herbal medicines 126
Oral contraceptive 7, 120
    pill 66, 69, 70, 79, 117, 145
        role of 70
Outflow obstruction 21
Ovarian cancer 12
Ovarian endometrioma 15, 28, 28*f*, 46, 51,
        54, 82, 83
    management of 98
Ovarian endometriosis 34, 47
    diagnosis of 10
Ovarian endometriotic cyst walls,
        laparoscopic excision of 40
Ovarian fossae, peritoneum of 12
Ovarian implants, morphology of 14
Ovarian microendometrioma 102
Ovarian preservation 74
Ovarian rupture 46
Ovarian torsion 46
Ovariectomy 97

EU GSPR Authorised Reprsentative
Logos Europe, 9 rue Nicolas Poussin
1700, La Rochelle, France
Phone: +33 (0) 6 67 93 73 78
E-mail: contact@logoseurope.eu

www.ingramcontent.com/pod-product-compliance
Ingram Content Group UK Ltd.
Pitfield, Milton Keynes, MK11 3LW, UK
UKHW051952240426
470334UK00003B/20